Living with a Spinal Cord Injury

Joseph English was living his best life when a car accident changed everything. He suffered life changing injuries, and the doctors told him there was no chance of recovery. Facing life as a quadriplegic, Joe lost his business, his romantic partner, and, for a while, his will to carry on. His story, told with extensive contributions from his family and friends, charts his journey from being dead at the roadside to finding something to live for as he recounts his progress from injury to survival.

With absolute candour, Joe tells the whole story of his accident, his rehabilitation, and his recovery. Full of advice and suggestions from professionals in the rehabilitation journey, this book is remarkably frank about the struggles Joe has endured, and the times when he felt as if life wasn't worth living. It addresses all the most difficult issues around life after paralysis, including loss of identity and letting go of the past, as well as providing practical information on topics such as assistive technology, financial claims, and legal support. It also outlines the various roles of those in the rehabilitation team. His doctors and specialist practitioners give their unique perspectives into their processes and procedures, helping to demystify them, while Joe's family and friends ask the kinds of questions readers will be asking too, making this an invaluable guide to what to expect for anyone going through a similar experience. The book shows – by lived example – that there is always more to live for.

It is essential reading for those with paraplegia, quadriplegia, and other spinal injuries, and their families, friends, and care-givers. It is also valuable for neuropsychologists, neurologists, and other rehabilitation therapists, as well as students in medicine, nursing, allied health, and neuropsychology.

Joseph English is a quadriplegic, paralysed from the neck down who suffered a life-changing car accident in his mid-twenties. Joe now fronts his own charity: Quad-Rebuild, which is gaining momentum.

After Physical Injury: Survivor Stories

Living with a Spinal Cord Injury
My life as a Quadriplegic
Joseph English

Living with a Spinal Cord Injury

Cord Injury

My life as a Quadriplegic

Joseph English

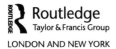
Routledge
Taylor & Francis Group

LONDON AND NEW YORK

Designed cover image: Joseph English

First published 2024
by Routledge
4 Park Square, Milton Park, Abingdon, Oxon OX14 4RN

and by Routledge
605 Third Avenue, New York, NY 10158

Routledge is an imprint of the Taylor & Francis Group, an informa business

© 2024 Joseph English

British Library Cataloguing-in-Publication Data
A catalogue record for this book is available from the British Library

ISBN: 9781032554419 (hbk)
ISBN: 9781032554402 (pbk)
ISBN: 9781003430728 (ebk)

DOI: 10.4324/9781003430728

Typeset in Times New Roman
by codeMantra

Contents

Contributors

Andy (Mentor Support)

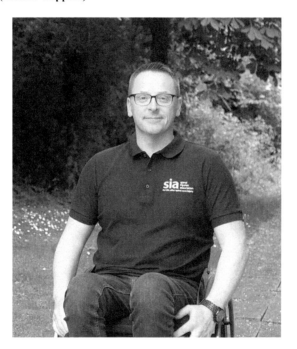

I am spinal cord injured myself; I sustained an injury to my back through a fall 20 years ago. I am a paraplegic, full-time wheelchair user. I have a little bit of movement and a little bit of sensation below my level of injury but not enough to be able to walk. I had some very difficult, dark days for the first few years after my injury, but I consider myself very fortunate in getting to where I am now. I tried to return to my previous job in mechanical engineering, but wasn't able to reach the level of work I expected of myself, so I embarked on further studies to qualify as a fitness instructor, and I went from there to working in a mainstream gym. I seized on an opportunity to travel, to play, and coach sport. I met my partner who is now my wife, and I began to consider where my life would turn next. Twelve years after my injury, the job of Support Coordinator with the Spinal Injuries Association came up. It was a golden opportunity to start a career, using all of my knowledge and experience, so I jumped at the chance. All of the work I'd done, my volunteering, my sports, and my coaching all fed into the role, and I got the job.

I work across the North East and Northern regions, and there are people like me offering the same range of services throughout the country. You can find out how to contact your local provider on the Spinal Injuries Association (SIA) website: www.spinal.co.uk

Barry (Joe's Friend)

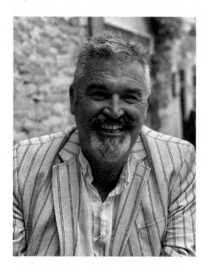

I had a business in Halifax, renovating and restoring old properties after fire and flood damage. It was quite a niche market, and I would be called in by insurance companies to make repairs for some high net-worth clients. The artisans I used had to be the best of the best, people I could trust. I was a member of the West Riding Stone Carving Association when Joe joined. Following in his father's footsteps, he thought he was already a pretty competent stone mason and wasn't bashful about saying so. He thought he'd inherited the skill through his bloodline. Joe told me a bit about the kinds of work that he did, and I kept him in the back of my mind in case we could work together in the future. A few months later, I got a job and invited Joe to get involved. He worked for me, and he did a really good job. After that we got to know each other better and better.

Carolyn (Serious Injury Solicitor)

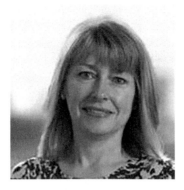

I'm a partner in the Complex Personal Injury team of national law firm, Irwin Mitchell LLP, and have specialised in brain and spinal cord injury claims for the last 28 years. I head the specialist neuro (brain/spinal) team in Leeds, and we often deal with very complex and highly fought claims involving substantial sums of money. We have three main aims: (1) to try and ensure our clients have access to first-class rehabilitation so they can have the best life possible after their accidents, (2) to secure our clients' financial future so they can pay for the things they now need because of their injuries, and (3) to provide a first class service to our clients.

Gez (Carer)

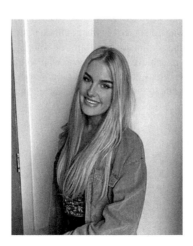

I was only due to stay for a few weeks, but ended up staying for a year and a half! I enjoyed getting to know Joe, we're of a similar age and we got on well. I provided day-to-day care for Joe, helping him to do some of the things he couldn't do on his own.

Hayley (Personal Assistant)

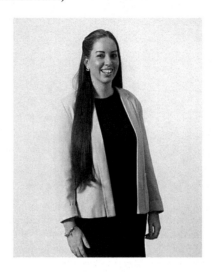

From the start, I could see that Joe was very driven. I found him honest and outspoken too; passionate about a lot of things, which all helped keep him going. Joe's will and his self-belief are incredibly strong, and they have allowed him to achieve so much, but I know it has been frustrating for him at times not to be able to do everything that he wants to do as easily as other people can. He recognised that he needed help with many of the practical elements of his life, so I help him achieve the things he wants to achieve.

It was clear that he wanted someone who could do more for him than handle his correspondence and administer his affairs, he wanted someone to help him drive what he wants to achieve, and someone who would share in his values and enthusiasm to get things done. My background was in charity and events work so I have been able to give him that peer-level support.

John (Chartered Financial Planner)

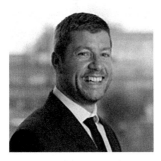

I am a Chartered Financial Planner at IM Asset Management Limited, part of the Irwin Mitchell Group. After graduating in 2000, I started working in Financial Services. In 2005, I travelled around the world, and on my return became a Financial Planner. I joined IM Asset Management in 2013, and specialise in providing financial advice to the recipients of substantial Personal Injury Settlements working alongside Deputies, Professional Trustees, and claimants' families. My role is to make sure clients have what monies they need year on year whilst achieving capital growth to fund future expenditure.

Kate (Joe's Friend)

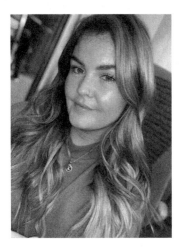

We've been friends for years. We're the same age and we were in the same year at high school, so we've been in each other's lives in some way since we were 11-years old. Our friendship really took off when we were around 12 or 13, and we went out as boyfriend and girlfriend for a few months. That didn't last, but it didn't stop our friendship, and we've been close ever since. We remained friends after high school, and we were in the same friendship group. I heard about Joe's accident while I was travelling, and it was a shock to see him when I got back. But seeing the change in him since then has been incredible.

Katherine (Neuropsychologist)

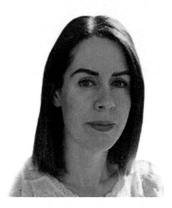

As a neuropsychologist I work with individuals who have been diagnosed with some form of acquired brain injury or neurological condition. I work very closely with families and care staff so that I can implement a bespoke plan of intervention to be carried out in close conjunction with other members of the team. I work a lot with case managers and rehab teams in situations where a client's funding comes from an insurance company. I also provide community rehabilitation to individuals who have been referred to the team by the NHS.

In my role I'm particularly concerned with the link between what has happened in someone's brain and any changes in thinking and memory, emotions and mood, and behaviour. I also work with my clients to understand the meaning of any traumatic event and how an individual now views themselves, others, and the world around them.

Katie (Senior Case Manager)

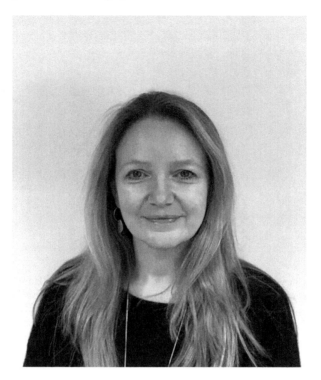

I'm an Occupational Therapist, and started my professional journey at the Princess Royal Spinal injury unit as a junior and senior OT. I've gained a wide range of experience of working with spinal cord-injured clients from both an OT and a care perspective. I worked for a large care company for a number of years, setting up care packages and supporting clients and the care team within the clients' own homes. Then I began working with Glynis Kenny, the founder of Spinal Injury Case Management Ltd., based in Wakefield, in 2012. In 2016 I was nominated for the CMSUK Case Manager of the year award. I'm proud that I can think of every one of my clients over the years, and know that I have been able to bring them positive change and support.

Mary (Joe's Mum)

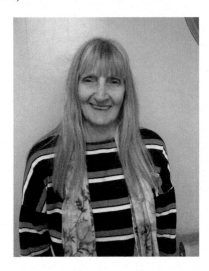

Joe was the youngest in the family and his brothers and sisters used to spoil him rotten! He was a clever lad – always taking things apart to see how they worked, and then reconstructing them. He was very particular about things, even his food. When he had beans on toast, he always used to cut his toast into triangles and then have the beans in the middle. Even after everything that has happened to him, I know he will be successful in his business. He's already done so many things the doctors said he'd never be able to do. He won't ever be left on his own. Even if it isn't me, or it isn't his dad, this family will be there for him.

Michaela (Joe's Sister)

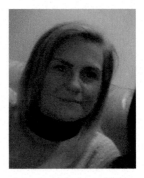

I'm 15 years older than Joe, so I used to babysit him sometimes, and take him to school. We had a good relationship growing up, we went on family holidays and spent a lot of time together. His accident was absolutely devastating, but we have all stuck together. If we're going out as a family now, we need to make sure things are disabled friendly, but apart from that, you'd think we were a pretty normal lot. It wouldn't have seemed possible a few years ago, but "the O'Shameless family" is back! (It can get quite loud and boisterous when we're all together!)

Paul (Joe's Brother)

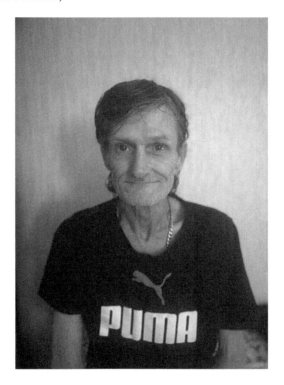

I'm quite a bit older than Joe, but we had a good relationship growing up. My mum and his dad were together at the time, and we saw each other nearly every day. We're quite different. He's always been such a grafter, and I'm a bit lazier than that! We're totally opposite in a lot of ways. When Joe was banned from driving, he used to ask me to help him out with the driving. He never would have thought about driving while he was banned, so I helped him for a few months. In spite of everything that's happened to him, Joe is strong, and he has never ever given up on himself.

Peter (Joe's Dad)

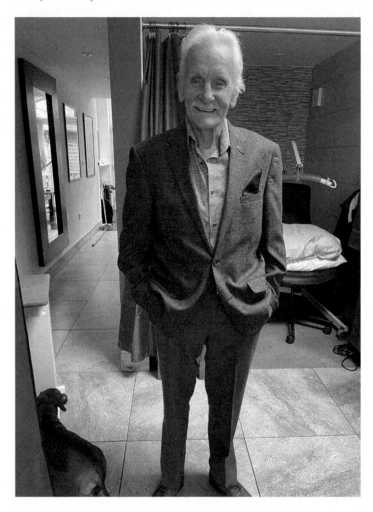

Joe learnt his trade with me, and I could see he had it in him to be successful. We have spent a lot of time together over the years – he has come back to live with me a few times, and when he was in hospital in Leeds, we drew up plans for an extension to my house so he could move in with me. We bounce off each other a bit sometimes, but we didn't want him moving into a care home. That wouldn't have been the right place for him. Joe then designed his own home, and the two of us have recently moved in there.

Rachael (Neuro Physiotherapist)

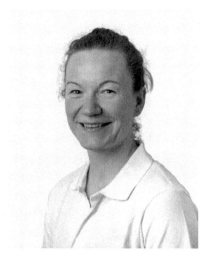

I'm part of a team of specialist neuro physiotherapists who work across a large population, primarily working with people with acquired neurological conditions, whether that's a result of a trauma, stroke, or other acquired impairment. The work that we do is partly around maximising independence, while also making sure that people remain healthy. I work for a company called Motion Rehab, and we provide a range of traditional physiotherapy, as well as a specialism in accessing technology.

Rohit (Spinal Injuries Consultant)

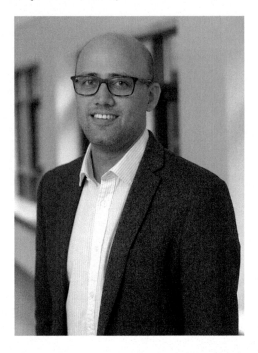

I'm a Spinal Injuries consultant, based at the Princess Royal Spinal Cord Injuries Centre, Northern General Hospital, Sheffield. There are only eight spinal cord rehab centres across England, and Sheffield is the second largest.

I did my initial training in India, where I did a degree and post-graduate training in Physical Medicine and Rehabilitation. That was followed by a two-year fellowship in spinal cord injury and musculoskeletal rehabilitation in Toronto, Canada. I came to Sheffield to undertake further training in spinal cord rehab, and then took up my consultant post in 2017. Joe was one of my first patients as consultant. It felt as if we were both going through our own learning experiences at that time.

Ross (Joe's Friend)

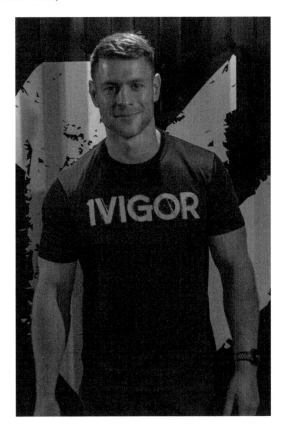

I was friends with one of Joe's best friends, and that's how I knew of Joe. I really started to get to know him properly at my stag do in 2013, and he was wild! He drank pretty much non-stop that day, and by the night he just decided he'd had enough, and he found his way home to Halifax from Essex. We didn't hear from him again for a week after that! I think he had a bit of a reputation for getting a bit wild on nights out. He was definitely a good laugh. But that wasn't all there was to Joe. Hardworking, helpful, and he'd do anything for a friend. He was a really nice bloke. He still is.

Sam (Joe's Sister)

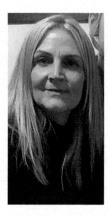

The one word that sums up what Joe was like is 'driven'. He was always working hard to make a success of everything he did. He started out watching his dad, and then picked it all up himself. He seemed to learn really quickly, and worked so hard at everything he did. His business was his life. Even when he wasn't working Joe would be keeping busy with something to keep his mind active. He was never one for sitting around idly doing nothing. He never even seemed to sleep much! He was always up early, and off and away to do something or other, and even now, he's full of ambition.

Samantha (Dietitian)

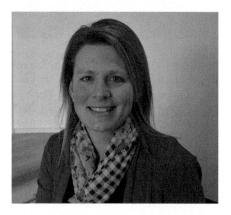

I'm a Dietitian and part of my role is supporting people like Joe to optimise their health through good nutrition. I studied nutrition and dietetics at university, and am registered with the HCPC – the health and care professions council. To remain on the HCPC register Dietitians are required to renew their registration every two years and we have to maintain continuous professional development. After my training, I worked clinically in the NHS for eight years in a variety of roles, one of which was on the intensive care unit. I also looked after a lot of children and young people with brain injuries and lifelong limiting conditions, some of whom where tube-fed, and some were fed orally. I now run a private practice and support people with acquired brain and spinal injuries. I really enjoy being able to work with people in their own homes, meet their families and support workers and provide a really tailored dietetic service.

Sean (IT Technician)

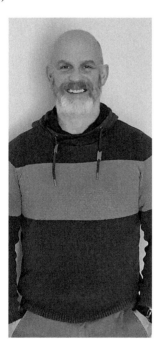

In 2005, I started working as an IT technician at a school for children with cerebral palsy, run by SCOPE. It was my job to help the pupils get the most out of the available technology so that they could get the most out of the curriculum. Before the school unfortunately closed down in 2010, I went part time and set up on my own. I had seen how technology frightened a lot of people that it was intended to help, including people with disabilities and their careers. I knew there was a wealth of technology out there to help and support them, but they weren't getting access to it, partly because they didn't know about it, or they didn't think they would be able to use it effectively, or because it was prohibitively expensive. I equipped myself with the basics and took myself out on the road looking to bring the technology to the people who needed it, and I was soon able to turn it into a full-time business.

Introduction

One mistake can change a life. In this book, I'm going to tell you about the mistake that turned my life upside down. More importantly, I'm going to tell you how I made the journey from living a 'normal' life to accepting and appreciating a very different life.

If you have sustained an injury that has left your body broken, and your spirit weak, this book is for you. This book is designed to help shape and develop your own thoughts on how you are going to live the rest of your life. I have experienced some of the lowest lows I think anyone can experience. I have felt that life was not worth living, and I have wanted to die. And yet, I have come out the other side, stronger in so many ways. People are right when they say, "time heals old wounds," and as time has gone on, I have found strength I didn't know I had. And I believe that you can too.

If you are the friend or loved one of somebody who is undertaking this journey, this book is for you too. No one ever knows what questions to ask somebody in my position, or how inquisitive they're able to be. This book will answer some of those questions for you and help you as you start to navigate a new life.

Before going into the details surrounding his accident in the following chapters, Joe and his family and friends discuss the boy he was, and the young man he had grown into before the crash. As the youngest in a large family, Joe's mother reveals that he was clever, but spoilt rotten as a child. Joe admits that, from a very young age, he was fascinated by how things worked, and used to spend many hours taking things apart. Joe is candid about some difficult times in his youth, but after being kicked out of school at 15, he went on to settle down and find his place in life. Everyone speaks of his skills as a stonemason, and his enthusiasm for his craft. And Joe's enthusiasm for stone carving and his drive to success in business set him on a course as a successful young man in his field.

Prologue

Who Was Joe English?

Joe:

Before I tell you my story, and talk about who I am, I'll let some of the people who know me best, sketch in some of the details of who I was…

Peter (Joe's Dad):

He was always building, and in some way, he always will be building. He went to work with me when he was just seven. By the time he was nine, I used to give him pieces of stone to work with and he could carve house numbers into them beautifully. He asked me how much he should charge, and I said £3 a letter, and he was quite pleased with that until I said, "What about the cost of the stone?" He got thrown out of school at 15, but he already knew he wanted to be a stone mason.

He did some work for me while he was doing his college course, and the college inspectors used to come out and check on his work. One day, they looked at a wall he'd built, and they were very happy with it. But I told them to look at it again, "What's wrong with that wall?" I asked. They looked again, and said, "It's very nice, very straight. I told them to look at the corners" He'd run out of bonding, and they hadn't noticed. Just as well I was there to point it out! He probably lost a few marks that day.

Paul (Joe's brother):

Even though I was a few years older than him, we had a good relationship growing up. My mum and his dad were together at the time, and we saw each other nearly every day. We're quite different. He's always been such a grafter, and I'm a bit lazier than that! We're totally opposite in a lot of ways. But everyone loved Joe. We still do.

Joe:

I am the youngest sibling out of twelve, with one real sister and eleven half brothers and sisters, but I class them all as my own. But while I am the youngest, I sometimes feel like the oldest.

Mary:

He was the youngest in the family and his brothers and sisters used to spoil him rotten! He was a clever lad – always taking things apart to see how they worked, and then reconstructing them. He was very particular about things, even his food. When he had beans on toast, he always used to cut his toast into triangles and then have the beans in the middle.

Joe:

Perhaps I *was* a bit spoilt growing up. I'll let the rest of my family confirm or deny that! I was very motivated to take things apart and build them up again. But it's fair to say that I went through some turbulent times, and I ended up being kicked out of school at 15. It wasn't the best time of my life, but even then, I had good friends, and I still had big ambitions.

Kate (Joe's Friend):

Seven or eight of us would go out together when we were old enough to go out drinking and partying. Joe partied hard. He had his wild years. He was the one who was always trying to get us to go out partying, but he was always a really hard worker too.

Joe:

I did party hard back then, and I lost myself for a few years. But I found my way back to where I wanted to be; I'd always had the idea of working in the building trade, and a love of stone masonry was already deeply ingrained; I already knew that's what I wanted to do.

I really settled down around the age of 20, when I met my partner at the time, and I set up as a sole trader with the aim of building up a client base. I loved it, and I was extremely dedicated about the work. I was fascinated by architecture and passionate about stonemasonry.

Barry (Joe's Friend):

Joe worked for me on and off, and we became really good friends. I liked Joe, I liked his work, and I liked the way he went about things. It took a while; Joe wasn't the easiest person to get to know and to like, he was always one for effing and jeffing, and I used to have to tell him to stop it sometimes, but over those few years, he became like a son to me.

Relationships between blokes tend to fall into different categories. Some blokes just want to bullshit you, tell you what they've done, and how good they are at everything. Joe had all the lip and the enthusiasm, but he was honest too. I could never have told him where he was going wrong with his costings, unless he'd had the humility to ask me, and he did. It felt like a son coming to his father for a bit of advice.

There was a major stone carving competition in Freiburg in Germany and Joe wanted to go. The problem was he didn't have any money. Back then Joe was living hand-to-mouth. He'd get a job, price it wrong, pay his lads, and have nothing left at the end of it. But Joe wasn't the kind of person who would listen if you tried to tell them where he was going wrong. I knew how keen he was to go, and I thought he'd probably do pretty well too.

I saw something in him, and I knew how much it meant to him. His enthusiasm was infectious, he didn't know when to stop sometimes! He'd take on far too much work, and try to please all the people all of the time. The only time I saw that boundless enthusiasm dashed when he told me he couldn't afford to go. I felt like he needed that opportunity, so I told him he was going, and I gave him the money. So off he went and won it. He won the top apprentice award for a bear scratching his back against a tree!

Joe:

I went to stone carving events every year, and I came first in that apprentice class in the 2014/2015 event Barry mentioned, for carving this bear...

I was building up a wealth of knowledge and experience that enabled me to land some good clients. I was very dedicated to the work. I loved it so much, I loved creating and crafting, and showing people what I could do, so I didn't see work as work. Even in my time off, I'd be going to look at buildings or working on some new stonemasonry or carving project of my own.

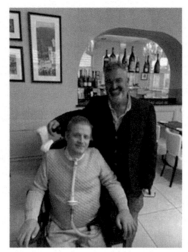

Joe and Barry

Kate (Joe's Friend):

> I went away travelling for a while, we still kept in touch. Joe seemed to have his life pretty sorted. He was doing so well at his stonemasonry, and I could see how hard he was working at his business. While I was away, I know he was constantly engaged in building up the business. He spent pretty much all of his time working. We met up again when I came back from travelling and he was still so focussed on growing his business. He was set on building a good life for himself.

Ross (Joe's Friend):

> I used to own a fencing company, and any time I needed help, Joe would be there, even though he had his own business to worry about. He didn't ask for any money, he didn't want anything for it. He was just happy to help. And when I did a full renovation on my house, and we were behind schedule he'd be there – ten o'clock at night – after he'd done a full day at work. And he'd be there, working away for me until the early hours. He wasn't there because he thought he had to be, you could tell he genuinely wanted to help.

Joe:

> I met Michelle in 2016, when I was 26, and we were in a relationship when the crash happened. It was love at first sight. She was an architect, so she could really relate to me. We were both

hardworking and driven, but we went on lots of holidays together. We were best friends, we loved going to new places to look at architecture, and we were always there for each other.

I didn't have time to take any time out of work back then. As well as all the work and the holidays, I got together with a couple of mates to invest in land that we could develop. We went to look at plots and had to work out how much each one would take to develop into something and see what we could make on one versus another to try to make the best possible profit margins. I was routinely doing 16–18-hour days at that point. I had up to 15 lads working for me throughout West Yorkshire.

I was advertising my services as a specialist stonemason and building contractor, and I was working hard to make us a cut above the rest, priding ourselves on our good company image and our sound environmental credentials. It was all building up, I was working until one in the morning, then going home for a few hours' sleep before getting up at six and starting all over again. I was burning the candle at both ends. But my course was set. I knew where life was taking me, and I could see my future with Michelle all mapped out in front of us. Or so I thought.

Barry (Joe's Friend):

When I had an extension built at home, I asked Joe to come and built it. And then he built another one for me, and just as he was finishing the second extension, the accident happened…

Part 1

The Accident and the Aftermath

1 Dead at the Roadside

It felt like just another day for Joe English, but this was the day when everything changed.

I remember hearing the crunch... and when I looked over, I saw Joe lying next to me. His leg was wrapped around the steering wheel, and he was absolutely still. He hadn't been wearing his seatbelt.

Joe:

I was up at six o'clock, as usual. It was a Sunday morning, but that didn't matter, work didn't stop for weekends. I was only in my mid-20s, but I was already a man on a mission; living life in a hurry. My whole future was mapped out in front of me: build up the business, get married, have kids, retire early, and enjoy life. I had my work, I had my family, and I had my soul mate, Michelle. Life was good.

With the business doing so well, I'd enjoyed some of the trappings of success and got myself a BMW 135 series car. I'd been a bit of a boy racer behind the wheel, flying up and down West Yorkshire, managing all my various projects. Full disclosure: I was caught speeding one too many times, and banned from driving for 18 months. (That car really did go very fast!) So, I employed my brother, Paul, to drive me about. I was supposed to be more of an office person, staying on top of all the quotes, plans, and contracts, as well as the tenders for Council work that had started trickling in. But if a project fell behind, or if the team needed my advice, I'd step in and help out. I needed someone who could be on hand at a moment's notice to take me wherever I needed to go, and Paul fit the bill. They were long days for both of us. If I got up at six, Paul needed to get up at six so he could drive me around. And if I finished at midnight – or more likely, after midnight – so did he.

DOI: 10.4324/9781003430728-2

Paul (Joe's Brother):

We'd started quite early for a Sunday, but that wasn't unusual for Joe, and I'd already taken him to quite a few places. He'd been planning to spend most of the afternoon in his office, so I dropped him off and waited to hear when I should pick him up and take him home. But then, halfway through the afternoon, he called and asked me to take him to look at some land he was interested in buying. I picked him up, and we drove an hour or so out towards Todmorden.

I'm older than Joe, and we had a pretty good relationship growing up, but there was something we argued about almost every time he got in the car; I would never set off driving until he'd put his seatbelt on, and there were a few times when I had to wait for Joe to buckle up.

Joe:

Paul was always telling me "You need to wear your seatbelt." But I was usually working on my laptop, or trying to sort out my paperwork, and it used to get in the way. I suppose I was a bit ignorant – maybe even a bit arrogant – but I'd never seen any safety campaigns or heard any horror stories about people not wearing their seatbelts.

I just remember being very tired that afternoon, and I know I must have drifted off, with my head against the passenger side door.

Paul (Joe's Brother):

It was getting on for late afternoon by the time we were heading back, and the light was already fading. I remember driving through Selby Bridge, I remember taking a couple of tight corners, carrying on down a straight road, and then...

We're still not sure how it happened. Joe was drifting in and out of sleep, and I think I must have nodded off too. I remember hearing the crunch, but that's all I can remember about the crash, until I woke and realised with horror that the van was on its side. We think the van hit the central reservation and then smashed into a tree on the pavement. I was still strapped in, but when I looked over, I saw Joe lying next to me. His leg was wrapped around the steering wheel, and he was absolutely still. I knew then that he hadn't been wearing his seatbelt.

I'd been so careful – I was always so careful. Joe used to say I mithered him about it all the time, but at some point on the journey, Joe must have taken his seatbelt off, and I didn't realise. I only wish I'd known. I could have stopped the car and made him put it back on.

I could feel pain in my ribs on the left-hand side of my body, and there was a little bit of blood, but I was otherwise okay. In the distance, I could hear the sound of the sirens coming towards us.

I managed to get out of my seat, and I wanted to get Joe out. I managed to pull his leg from around the steering wheel, and pull him straight so I could support his head in my hands. He was trying to tell me something, but I couldn't quite work it out. It was either 'I can't move,' or 'I can't breathe…'

I wanted to get him out of the van, but as I tried to start dragging him to safety, a firefighter shouted at me to leave him where he was. There were voices all around us then, and someone else said, "He's not breathing!" That's when everything changed, and we had to get him out of the van as quickly as possible. One of the firemen brought him round and got him breathing again. But for those few minutes, he was dead.

They had Joe stretched out on the road. There were emergency services personnel everywhere. They worked on getting a line in him, and all the while it was getting darker and colder and harder for them to work.

Michaela (Joe's Sister):

I was at work when I got the call… I asked someone to cover for me for half an hour, never in a million years expecting the extent of what I was about to see. When I got there, it was carnage. There were fire engines, ambulances, and police; the road was completely blocked off and I thought the worst. Someone told me they were waiting for an ambulance to take Joseph to Leeds. I knew it was bad then, but I could never have expected it to be as bad as it really was.

Paul (Joe's Brother):

Eventually, they got him into the air ambulance and took him to Leeds. They checked me over at the roadside and then put me in an ambulance. At the hospital, they listened to my heart and checked my ribs, and put a collar on me to help with the whiplash. I still didn't know what had happened to Joe. I didn't even know if he was still alive.

Mary (Joe's Mum):

Getting the phone call from Joe's girlfriend, Michelle, was one of the worst things that you can imagine. She said they'd cut Joe out of the van and taken him to Leeds in the air ambulance. None of us really knew how it had happened. To this day, I still don't know exactly how it happened. I know you can see it all happening on the dashcam video, but I can't watch it. I've never been able to watch it, and I don't think I ever will.

There were so many what-ifs… What if Joe had been wearing his seatbelt… What if he'd done what he'd planned to do that day, and just stayed in his office that afternoon... All I know for sure is that poor Paul blamed himself. It was a horrendous time for all of us, but it was especially hard for him.

We rushed to the hospital not knowing if Joe would still be alive when we got there.

Joe:

I don't remember any of it. I can look at the video and see that it's me, but I don't remember any of it happening to me. The first thing I do remember is waking up in intensive care, not knowing where the hell I was. I looked around the room and Paul was sitting there. He just kept saying, "I'm sorry, bro! I'm sorry!"

2 The Decision to Live or Die

Joe's family and friends share their experiences of the first few days after the accident, and Joe begins to realise the full extent of his injury.

I'd never, ever, seen my dad cry, until I saw him crying by the side of my bed in intensive care.

Sam (Joe's Sister):

The phone rang in the middle of the night. You always know it's bad news when that happens. It was Michaela calling to tell me that Joe had been in a really bad accident. She said he was in a coma, and they didn't think he was going to survive.

Paul (Joe's Brother):

When they tried to get him out of the coma, Joe was so disorientated, and so upset – he just didn't know what was happening to him – so they had to put him straight into an induced coma. Later, he told me that he thought he'd been flying about with monks, and there were other hallucinations too; frightening, nightmarish things.

Joe:

It's hard to look back on that experience in intensive care. The one thing I remember most was waking up and seeing my dad. I'd never, ever seen my dad cry, until I saw him by the side of my bed in intensive care. But I don't remember much else. I was heavily sedated, and it felt like I was in a hallucinogenic state. Part of me felt like I could hear people who had died. They were saying things like "I'm sorry, Mum. You'll see me again one day." Other times, I felt like I was lost in a nightmare and couldn't find my way out.

All they told my family when I was taken in was, "Let's just see if he makes it through the first twenty-four hours," but the expectation was that I wouldn't. Even if I did, they said I would be so severely brain damaged, my family would have a decision to make: should

DOI: 10.4324/9781003430728-3

they keep my ventilator going and keep me alive, or switch it off and let me die.

Sam (Joe's Sister):

When we were finally allowed to see him, he was still in the induced coma. Even though we'd been told what to expect, walking into that room was horrible. I couldn't ever have prepared myself for seeing him like that, covered in all those tubes and wires.

Paul (Joe's Brother):

It was a horrible time. It was at least a week until I got to saw Joe again. At first, they were really only letting Joe's girlfriend, Michelle, in to see him, and maybe they didn't think I was ready to see him again after what had happened. It was so frustrating not seeing him, and I felt like I didn't know what was going on. It was only later that I found out they'd given him just 24 hours to live. I'm not sure how I'd have coped if I'd known that at the time.

Michaela (Joe's Sister):

When I saw him in the resus room in Leeds General Infirmary, it was so strange. There were tubes everywhere, but he didn't look to have a single bruise on his body. I couldn't help thinking *it can't be that bad, surely?* I just didn't know how severe his internal injuries were. When we learned just how significant it was, we knew we had to prepare for the worst, and that's what I had to tell people on the phone.

Somehow, Joe clung onto life, and when the 24 hours had passed, it felt like maybe he was through the worst of it. But it wasn't that simple. That's when they told us that even if he did survive – and it was still a big if – he'd have no quality of life. He wouldn't be able to talk, he wouldn't be able to eat. He would be paralysed and on a ventilator for the rest of his life. There wasn't any doubt in their minds that his life was practically over.

In those first few days, we all did more crying than anything else. The shock of it was awful. And the questions that came with it were horrible too. On the one hand we were praying for him, saying you're strong Joe, you can get through this. But on the other hand, with everything the doctors were telling us, we thought you are not going to want to live like this. Selfishly we wanted him to stay with us, but we had to consider that he might not want to.

Mary (Joe's Mum):

Eventually, they brought him round from the induced coma very gradually so they could help him understand where he was, and what had happened. Michelle was with him for those first few days, but they wouldn't let anyone else see him, so we had to rely on her reports. It was terrible not knowing what was happening hour by hour. But when we did get to visit him, the things that we saw in there really affected us. I was numb with shock, we all were.

Barry (Joe's Friend):

It was family only at first, and it was horrible not being able to see him. I know that his mum never left. She practically slept on a chair in the room. My wife and I had got to know his girlfriend, Michelle, quite well; we'd spent lots of time with the two of them, and I had to rely on her to tell me what was going on. The news was all bad. There were so many bad nights when it seemed as if no one thought he was going to pull through. By the time I was allowed to go to Leeds, I was already thinking: is this the last time I'm going to see Joe?

I didn't know what to expect, and at first, all I could see was the tubes and wires. He looked as if he was at death's doorstep. It reminded me of the last time I saw my dad in hospital, and knowing he was close to death. Joe was unconscious, and with nothing to suggest he was ever going to come out of it, the sight of him lying there, being kept alive, stayed with me for days.

Ross (Joe's Friend):

I heard that he'd been in an accident through a friend. But at first, nobody really knew just how bad it was. It was a week afterwards that I heard just how bad his condition was. I saw him in intensive care a couple of times and that was hard, I was crying after that. Seeing him in that bed was so tough. And that's when it really hit home – this was serious. His family were hopeful of course, but we knew his outlook wasn't great, and the doctors were saying we have to be realistic about his chances.

Paul (Joe's Brother):

When I finally saw him, I couldn't stop crying. I just remember telling him over and over again that I was so sorry; how I would have swapped places with him if I could have. And I meant it. He was conscious, he knew I was there with him, but he couldn't speak. I came away from that first meeting more upset than I'd ever been, knowing that it was all my fault.

Barry (Joe's Friend):

One of the hardest things you might experience when you see a friend or loved one in that state is guilt. To see someone who has been so fit and healthy incapacitated like that can flick a switch inside you. When I saw Joe and I realised how badly he was hurt, and how much he was going to lose, I felt guilty. I think that's an understandable reaction.

Peter (Joe's Dad):

Once they'd stabilised him, they had to do an operation on his throat to put in a stoma. I had to give the consent for that, and I didn't know if I was doing the right thing, but we knew he wouldn't survive without it if they took him off the ventilator.

I thought he was through the worst of it after that, but the nurse told me he could still die at any minute. I thought he's always been an awkward little bugger, but he's going to have to be even more awkward to get through this.

Mary (Joe's Mum):

Because Joe wasn't able to talk after the accident, we didn't know what psychological state he was in, we didn't even know how badly his brain might have been damaged. They put an iron rod in his head to monitor his brain activity, but they were already telling us he would never be able to speak again, and he'd never be able to eat without being peg-fed.

Sam (Joe's Brother):

The doctors were brutally honest about his chances of recovery. When they talked to us about his prospects, it was clear that they were preparing us for the terrible decision Joe was going to have to make. Knowing that he would have to face such a stark choice between life and death was horrible. We all knew that if Joe's brain was working normally, but he was unable to do anything physically, there was a very real chance he would have chosen to end his life. It was a terrifying thought. But, knowing Joe like we did, we all felt that, as long as there was the slightest chance of life, Joe would take it, and he would do everything possible to make his recovery work.

We just had to stick together. We have always been a close-knit family. We've had our ups and downs like most families, but we have always been there for each other, no matter what. Those days were the hardest that our family have ever faced, knowing that even after he had survived the accident, we could still lose him.

Joe:

I spent seven weeks in intensive care, locked in my own mind, unable to speak, but slowly becoming more aware of my surroundings, even if I still didn't quite know what had happened. Michelle was in there with me in those first few days, weeks, and months. She took the time off work to be there by my side, and I think my feelings for her helped me make my decision to carry on. Even when I was oblivious to everything else, I could hear her voice reading to me. I couldn't quite work it out at the time, I didn't know why I could hear her, but I couldn't see her.

Michaela (Joe's Sister):

Thankfully, as the time wore on, we learned that his brain was working okay, and he started to show little signs that he might be making some kind of a recovery.

Mary (Joe's Mum):

After weeks of not knowing whether he could understand us, or communicate in any way, Joe started mouthing words. At first, he would get very frustrated that no one could understand him. It was horrible for him, feeling like he was locked in his own body, unable to reach out, unable to speak.

Joe:

When I tried to mouth words to people no one could really understand what I was trying to say, and I felt even more trapped in my body. The smallest tings are excruciatingly frustrating – imagine having an itch and not being able to scratch it. If you're a friend, relative, or carer of a quadriplegic, or someone who has been incapacitated by injury, I ask you to try it: the next time you feel an itch; see how long you can last without scratching it even as the urge to scratch builds up and up!

Sam (Joe's Sister):

You can imagine his frustration. Everything he wanted to do was difficult or impossible. He couldn't speak, so he used to make a noise with his lips and his tongue to try and get someone's attention. And that was the only thing he could do to show us he needed something. Imagine what it was like for him not even being able to scratch an itch. Just thinking about having an itch now is making me want to scratch. The part of his face that Joe could still feel was full of strange prickly sensations and itches and it used to drive him crazy.

But the fact that he was trying to communicate was so important. That's when we could tell that Joe was still in there. He had capacity, and he would be able to take ownership of the decision the doctors had been preparing us for…

Mary (Joe's Mum):

> Michelle was there for him, and she started to lip read for him. She was one of only a few people who could understand what he was trying to say.

Joe:

> Michelle was the only one who could lip read exactly what I wanted to say. Not even the nurses could do it, and the horror of having an itch and desperately wanting someone to scratch it, but not being able to communicate it used to drive me mad. Was that what my life was going to be like?

Mary (Joe's Mum):

> From a doctor's point of view, Joe didn't really have a future. They told us we would have to let him decide if he wanted to go on living or not... and we would have to live with whatever choice he made.

Michaela (Joe's Sister):

> By that stage it was clearly understood that Joe would need medical attention and treatment for the rest of his life, that he would most likely never walk, talk, or eat again, and it would be up to him to decide whether he wanted to live a 'reduced' life or not. Joseph could have given in, and no one would have blamed him for that. But it was so hard for all of us knowing that he could have been so close to making a decision to end his life.

Barry (Joe's Friend):

> Joe had been dead at the roadside. They'd had to bring him back to life two or three times, and I think about what I would have wanted... Would I have wanted to come back after that? None of us can imagine what it's like to lose everything you've got; to lose all your capability and end up being totally reliant on someone else.
>
> He needed a machine to breathe for him. It was classified as an invasive machine, and it meant that Joe could have gone through channels to request to have that machine removed. He would have been dead in 15 minutes. I kept going back to that thought – knowing that he had it in his power to turn the machine off, and I wondered what I would have done.
>
> Somehow, we had to leave all of that at the hospital door. Joe needed our support and encouragement.

Joe:

> Everyone seemed really cheery, and I later found out it was because all my visitors were under strict instructions not to cry around me. They were told to be as cheerful as possible so that I didn't get

anxious. I remember people stroking my hair and leaning in close to try and understand what I was attempting to say to them if I moved my mouth.

Ross (Joe's Friend):

When Joe was conscious enough to hear it – and they knew his brain was working – a doctor had that conversation with him and talked him through his chances of making any kind of recovery. It sounds harsh, but I think that really helped Joe. As much as it hurt, that was the point where he realised where he was, and he began to understand what his future might look like.

Before that, some people had been saying, you can go to Switzerland or America… they can do wonders out there, you can get the feeling back in your body. I'm not sure that helped. It gave Joe false hope; he was starting to imagine that he could feel things in his arms and the Doctor had to tell him that he really wasn't feeling anything. He *couldn't* feel anything. It was just his mind playing games with him. They'd seen that injury too many times and they knew he wasn't going to recover from it, not fully.

It must have been brutally hard for him to hear someone tell him he was going to be paralysed from the neck down for the rest of his life, but it cleared away the false hopes. He knew what his situation was then, and that horrible dose of reality really helped him focus on the truth of his situation.

After that, it was up to Joe to decide…

Joe:

I know my family talked about it and my dad told them to keep me alive. And then, when I was conscious, they had to ask me the same question: *do you want to live like this?* I can't really remember it clearly because it felt so weird and hallucinatory; but I know they laid it all out for me:

> The likelihood is that you will never be able to move, or speak, or eat, or do anything. You will be peg-fed for the rest of your life, and you will never be able to go anywhere or do anything without significant difficulty. You will never have the quality of life that you deserve.

They were preparing me for a life of misery, they were laying it all out so I could make my decision knowing the reality of what was waiting for me.

I didn't feel upset, but I was angry. *I felt: how can you tell me what I can and can't do in my life? How can you dictate what my life will be?* The decision hung over me…

On the day I had to decide, Michelle helped me to communicate my decision to my family: I said even if I don't move again, it doesn't mean that it will stop me achieving things. Everything the doctors said helped to spur me on. And it's strange, I think something changed in me. Before the accident, I had always been a bit of a pessimist. But the accident instilled a desire in me to do whatever I could do to get through it. Even then, I felt as if I wanted to prove to people that if I could do it, if I could move on from what had happened and start again, then they could do it too. There was some part of me that was refusing to give up. I didn't know – I couldn't know – what was waiting for me, I just knew I couldn't back down.

3   Seeing Red

Joe regains his voice, and begins to navigate the emotional aftermath of what has happened to him.

There were times when I couldn't face another hour, let alone another day, but somewhere deep inside, the sense of striving for a new destiny kept me going.

Joe:

While I was in intensive care, there were others; people like me who had been involved in dreadful accidents, people who couldn't move or do anything. I lay there, day after day, night after night, feeling like I never slept, just listening as hospital staff would ask those people, "Is there anyone there? Can you squeeze my hand if you can hear me?" I knew that's what had happened to me. I knew that's what my family had had to face, and I knew that some of those people would probably never recover. Some would leave the hospital in wheelchairs; some would never go home. Some of them didn't even last 24 hours.

Peter (Joe's Dad):

Eventually, they moved him out of that room onto a ward with more people. He was one of the lucky ones. That lad who was in there after him had been beaten up outside a nightclub; he was dead the next day. It was only really when he was with other people and starting to talk again that he really started to grasp what had happened to him.

Mary (Joe's Mum):

It was weeks till we heard his voice again. They'd inflated the balloon on the tracheostomy to ensure that no food could get into his lungs. When it was inflated, he had to be tube fed, and it wasn't until they started to let it down a little bit when his breathing was stronger, that he was able to try to speak again.

DOI: 10.4324/9781003430728-4

Michaela (Joe's Sister):

> The first time I heard his voice after the accident, I cried. It must have been four weeks since he'd been able to make any meaningful sound at all. They deflated the cuff on his ventilator and he made a low growling sound, but it was a huge step forward.

Mary (Joe's Mum):

> It was an amazing moment when he was able to talk to us again. After that, he started to eat again too, it was only soft foods at first because he had to learn how to swallow again. It was amazing for us to learn just how much the spine controlled everything. We had no idea.

Kate (Joe's Friend):

> It was after I'd gone travelling when he had his accident, and his world came crashing down. It was not long before I was due to come back, so he was still in hospital when I saw him. I went to see him with one of my other friends. He was asleep when we got there, and he had no idea that we were going to see him. When he woke, his face lit up. He still couldn't talk very well at that time, his voice was really quiet, but he was obviously so happy to see us.

Barry (Joe's Friend):

> After they deflated the cuff, allowing Joe to talk through his voice-box, it changed everything. At first it was wonderful to hear, but as Joe realised just how much his life had changed, he inevitably got more and more angry, and it came out in his words. The swearing started, and I knew that, for the family, it must have been hurtful and out of character; it wasn't a side of Joe that they had really seen before, and after the accident, it was running rampant.

Michaela (Joe's Sister):

> In the beginning, everything was impossible – and Joseph knows – he was awful to people. It wasn't the Joe we knew, but you can't be the same after an accident like that. It wasn't just the physical impact, the accident changed him as a person. It changed his personality. In the early days when he was in hospital, he could be nasty. He said some really horrible things to us. It took him some time to start to get past what had happened and what it had done to him.

Mary (Joe's Mum):

> He was horrendous in Sheffield. He would shout us out of the room every two minutes, telling us to F-off. It was upsetting and it was hard to hear, but I know it was more from frustration than anything else. And we could understand that.

Joe:

As everyone knows, those first few months, even years are horrible, but the first few weeks are close to being unendurable. Even though I made that decision to fight, it didn't make it any easier to come to terms with what had happened, and there were plenty of times when I felt like I had made the wrong decision. There were even times when I couldn't face another hour, let alone another day, but somewhere deep inside, the sense of striving for a new destiny to do something better kept me going, even when everything inside me was begging to give in.

Mary (Joe's Mum):

None of us could know just how hard it was for Joe, and we were frightened that at any moment, he might say he didn't want to be here anymore. We knew that there were times when he wanted to just let go. He was just so angry.

Michaela (Joe's Sister):

As a family we were there for him no matter what. Of course we were. And we knew it wasn't him when he lashed out. Not really. It was just what the accident had done to him. But there were many times when I walked out of hospital crying because he'd been mean and nasty to me.

I knew – and we all knew – that it was just his frustration. Whatever he wanted to do, he couldn't do. I can't imagine what that was like. To watch someone you love going though that is so hard, and I don't know how I would have coped with what he went through.

Barry (Joe's Friend):

What happened to Joe had an impact on all our lives. You're not trained to be able to deal with it, just as you, or your friend or loved one won't be trained in how to deal with it either if you're going through this now. You don't know what's going to happen in the days, weeks, months, and years ahead. You just have to try and adapt, and that isn't easy for anyone. Sadly, there will always be some friends and relatives who find that they just can't adapt, and those are the people that end up walking away. But some people empathise. They understand at least some of the difficulty that their friend is going through; they appreciate the depth of their friend's anger.

Joe:

No matter how hard it was for my family and friends, and how much harder I made it for them when I got angry, they were all there for me day after day. Even knowing I had their full support, I felt as if I was the furthest away from them that I had ever been. So much had changed. *Everything* had changed. In the first days and weeks, I literally couldn't communicate with them. Then, when I got my voice back, I still didn't feel like I could communicate with them in the way they wanted. I was just too volatile.

When people see you and you're beside yourself with rage and fury because of what's happened, they don't know how to deal with it. For most people it is a whole new experience. So how do you deal with someone you know and love when their anger has turned them into someone else? In my case, I feel as if the anger came from the control freak inside me. He had lost his grip on my life, and he didn't know how to deal with it.

Andy (Mentor Support):

It was still a little while before I would meet Joe, but I can say, from experience, that in the early days, the unknown is terrifying. You just don't know what is going to happen after a spinal cord injury and that fear can be hard to deal with. That inevitably triggers a lot of different responses in different people, and not all of them can be predicted by the type of person you know yourself to be. Some withdraw into themselves and stop speaking to others. Some lash out and get angry.

I was one of those people. I got quite angry, more at myself than anyone else. I am spinal cord injured; I sustained an injury to my back through a fall 20 years ago at the time of writing. I am a paraplegic, full-time wheelchair user. I have a little bit of movement and a little bit of sensation below my level of injury but not enough to be able to walk.

I had some very difficult, dark days for the first few years after my injury, but reflecting on what I have been through and where I am now, I consider myself very fortunate to have weathered the storm in getting to where I am now. I was aware that Joe was experiencing some of that anger too. I think it's important that people don't fixate on those reactions. It's how you come out of it that matters.

Sam (Joe's Sister):

Seeing him so frustrated and angry was one of the hardest things. Sometimes we had to leave him crying and feeling like the world was against him, and in those moments, there isn't much you can do. In those moments, there is nothing worse.

If you, your friend, or loved one is going through this, you're probably thinking *this is never, ever going to get any better.* You're probably asking all sorts of questions; you might even be asking: why me/why us? What have we done to deserve this? Stay strong. It might not seem like it, but it will get better.

Joe:

> It's okay to be angry. You have to allow yourself the time within your rehabilitation to accept those times when you might not have been a nice person. You can address them later, and you can apologise – if you need to – later.

Andy (Mentor Support):

> It's a long process, and if you're reading this early in your recovery, it will feel like an insurmountable mountain at times, and I urge you to learn how to be patient. I'll admit it, I struggled massively with that, and I could see the same impatience in Joe, and in so many others. It's natural. You want things to be done there and then. You want to be able to do things yourself, and you can't. That was the thing that brought the anger out in me. I couldn't do the things I wanted to do in the way I wanted to do them straightaway. I had to learn patience. You will too. And if that is still too difficult, there is counselling out there to help you. And there are people out there who will do their very best to support you through it.
>
> I will say that if there are specialist services available to you, whether that's psychology, counselling, or whatever, don't dismiss it. I did dismiss it at first. I didn't want any support from anyone, even people who had had similar injuries themselves. It was too soon for me, I didn't feel as if I related to those people. Looking back, I realised that I'd turned down so many things that could have been so helpful for me, and I thought, *what an idiot*! So I really do urge you to try and be open to at least speaking to people who can support you through the adjustment period and might have ways of helping you to cope with your anger.

Michaela (Joe's Sister):

> From our experience with Joe, we know you will face times when the anger and frustration threaten to overwhelm and take over. It's so hard, unbearably hard, not being able to do what you used to be able to do, or seeing a loved one struggling to do those things.
>
> If your friend or loved one is in that space now, if they are angry and lashing out, try and imagine what it must feel like not to be able to do any of the things you take for granted. Imagine how that must play on your mind. That's where I used to get my patience from.
>
> As a family we found that we shouldn't make too many allowances. As far as you can, you need to try and be normal with them. Yes, their life has changed, and yes, they definitely need your sympathy and understanding, but they don't need you to change who you are. That isn't going to help them in the long run.

Andy (Mentor Support):

It's that tacky old line, but time heals. It really does.

The longer that you are in this new situation that you have found yourself in, the easier it becomes. Day by day, week by week. In the early days, you're learning hour by hour. You're learning from every aspect of care that is provided, you're learning from every difficulty you have that you didn't have before, and you're learning how to do things for yourself in a different way. And just as importantly, you'll be learning how to ask for help to do things to enable you to do what you want to do.

Every aspect of care you receive helps you to adjust to the situation, and gives you the knowledge of how to go on and do these things yourself, or to be as independent as possible by guiding others to help you. Learning these things will help and enable you to live your life again.

Joe:

There will still be many times when you are not okay. And, even if you've heard it a hundred times, I'm going to say it one more time: it's okay not to be okay. Whatever is hurting you now, whatever is not okay for you, try to remember that it won't necessarily be like that forever. There are some things you won't be able to change, so you need to find a way to be kind to yourself. Some of that is about showing compassion to other people. But some of that is about showing compassion to yourself.

Everyone's experience is different. Depression, resignation, or a failure to accept what's happened can hit people extremely hard. But for me, it was anger, and it hit home as soon as I began to appreciate what had happened. I didn't want to have to listen to another person saying, "It's going to be okay." They were telling me you'll be able to work again, and all I could think in response was, "I've lost everything I've worked for, I've lost my company; you don't have a fucking clue."

In those days, and in the days that follow, you don't need someone to tell you things will get better, you just need someone to be there for you. It's not about the words. No words can describe what that kind of support means. You just need someone to be calm, to be a good listener, and to be there for you when you need them. It was like they said in hospital, if the people around you panic, it was only going to make me panic even more.

Andy (Mentor Support):

Joe has shown that you can come out the other side, you can leave that anger behind, and it will be wonderful when he has an opportunity to go back to Leeds and Sheffield to show some of those people just how far he has come. I think the people who helped him in those early days will be absolutely amazed. I think it's so important for as many people as possible who are involved in helping people through this to see the before and after. Too many of them see the anger and the pain and the confusion, but they don't get to see the man or woman on the other side of that. That's really important, I think, in spreading better understanding of how the process often works, particularly in Intensive Care and spinal units. It's just not possible to grasp quite what those people are going through. I'm so glad to have been a small part in that process with Joe, and everyone who gets involved can play their part too.

Joe:

Whether you're in my position, or you're a friend or loved one, this one tip above all others might just save your relationship! When the anger comes, it can sometimes be better for friends and loved ones to just leave. It's different for everyone of course, but for me, I just wanted people to say, "I'm here if you need me…" and then leave me to it. They came to understand that I was going to get angry sometimes. They knew it was okay for me to get angry, and I wasn't going to feel like that forever.

If you are visiting someone, you should know that your visits mean so much. So I urge you to try and let your loved one work through their anger, and most of all, try not to take it personally.

And if it's you in that bed, remember that most people will never have seen you like that before. So, they will need to adjust too. But trust them. Your real friends will keep coming back…

My best friend didn't come and see me for months. And when he did, I didn't want to know. I told him to get out of my fucking room. But he didn't. He sat there, and he took all the shit I had to give him, and at the end of the day, we were okay. There are not many people like that out there.

Barry (Joe's Friend):

I know it was tough for everyone who wanted to come and see him to make it. I hadn't long retired, so I was able to go and see Joe every day in the hospital in Leeds. I didn't ever want him to be on his own. We'd talk about any old shit really. Everyone I knew in the world of stone cutting knew Joe, and I had to give them daily updates on his progress. It was important to keep Joe abreast of their lives too, so that he still felt connected to the outside world.

Joe:

It was hard at first, but at some point, I did have to try and appreciate that what had happened to me had affected everyone else too. All my friends and family were struggling with what had happened. Strange as it was to admit, or accept, I wasn't the only victim.

Kate (Joe's Friend):

I used to get so upset after those early visits. It was heartbreaking seeing him like that. We all were. Inevitably, seeing someone so close to you in that situation can't help but make you feel grateful for whatever you've got in life. It was especially sad knowing how hard he'd been working, knowing that he hadn't seen as much of his friends as he would have liked over the last couple of years before the accident. He had put so much hard work into making his life a success and then he was told that he'd never be able to do any of those things ever again.

He was obviously very low for a very long time. There were times when he just didn't want to be here. He asked over and over, "Why has this happened to me?" It wasn't as if he was giving up, he just didn't know how to make his life work again. He thought his life was effectively over.

Sam (Joe's sister):

When this dreadful accident happened, we tried to find out as much as we could about the impact on Joe, and the likely outcomes for what he could achieve in the future, and I advise you to do the same. In the hospital, they gave us the worst-case scenario – and I understand why they need to do that – but it was important for us to find out what he might be able to do. Joe has achieved so many of the things they said he would never do. And because that happened to us, I really do say, don't give up hope.

Our attitude was let's just see. Take each day as it comes and deal with it, and don't put any limits on their future. I know there were times when it was too much for him. There were even times when he said he couldn't carry on. We used to say look how far you've come, look what you have already achieved in your recovery. One minute they were saying you'd never drink, eat, or speak, and now you're doing all those things, and more. Joe went from not being able to eat anything to eating ice cream, and that was one of the best sights of our lives.

Andy (Mentor Support):

If you're a friend or a loved one of someone who has been affected by this kind of injury, do remember there is help is out there for you too. You can get in touch with us at www.spinal.co.uk; we can provide specialist clinical support and advocacy for those who find themselves without the appropriate care or knowledge, provided by people like myself who have been through it. You can also contact Joe's own charity: Quad-Rebuild www.quad-rebuild.co.uk – he can put you in touch with people who will help to allay so many of your fears, and will help you all process the changes that have taken place. It's about looking forwards too, they will help you see what possibilities are still out there for you and for your family. We all have a fear of the unknown after an event like this, and the best people to help you are the ones that have been through it, or are going through it now. Whether you take away some reassurance, or some practical tips and advice you can use, they will help you massively.

4 Learning to Let Go of My Old Life

One of the hardest stages in anyone's recovery is trying to let go of the past. As Joe moved forwards in his recovery, the harsh reality of the life that lay ahead of him was growing clearer.

Before I thought about starting again, I had to come to terms with everything I had lost.

Michaela (Joe's Sister):

I tried, but I knew I couldn't ever imagine what Joe was going through. As a family, we all felt that sense of devastation, but it must have been a hundred times worse for him in adjusting to those new restrictions. Naturally, he was angry; he had worked so hard to get to where he was. He used to work such long hours. Even when he was out on a building site, he'd go home and do quotes for jobs until ten or eleven at night. He had been constantly on the go.

That accident took his life away. Everything that he knew, and everything that he was working towards was gone in an instant. How do you come to terms with that?

Katherine (Neuropsychologist):

For most people, one of the hardest steps along the road is accepting what has happened, without taking on any blame or guilt. Joe once told me that he cried for three to four months after the accident because he just wanted his old life back. But at the same time, he knew that had got him nowhere.

If you are going through an experience like Joe, it's important for you to know that reaching a place of acceptance for what has happened and what has been lost isn't going to feel like a switch turning on, but more of a gradual shift in your mindset…

Joe:

I was only at the start of my journey. At that time, my mindset was very firmly stuck. I still felt as if I was destined to be with Michelle.

DOI: 10.4324/9781003430728-5

I could see that the hard work I'd put into my business had started to pay off. I wasn't ready or prepared to let any of that go.

How do you move from thinking: my life is sorted, through to my life is in tatters, to finally emerging as a new man on the other side? I think perhaps that sometimes you have to look back to see where you've come from to see where you might be going. As my family tell the story, it seems as if I already had the strength and the skills I needed to start again. I just didn't know it yet...

Peter (Joe's Dad):

No one should have to go through what he had to endure, but if anyone could do it, Joe could. You could see the signs from an early age: the determination he needed to get through this.

Katherine (Neuropsychologist):

I know that many people are unable to contemplate life after an injury like the one Joe has suffered. Or start to think of themselves living a different kind of life. But having worked with so many people who have experienced significant and life-altering trauma, I have seen that people have a remarkable ability to adapt and move towards a place of change. Naturally, they can get stuck along the way, and that's when professional interventions can be helpful.

Mary (Joe's Mum):

It really helped him when he started talking to the psychologists, and after a while, he really wanted to see Paul.

Joe:

From a distance of five years, I know just how important talking is. I know it isn't always easy for us men to talk openly about our feelings for fear of being perceived as weak. But the only way you can really face your difficulties and start to come to terms with what you've lost is by taking about it. The alternative is that all those things just fester inside of you. Learning to talk openly takes time. But I promise you it is incredibly worthwhile.

Paul (Joe's Brother):

I still hadn't talked about the crash very much. Most people can't understand what it's like to go through something like that; you can only really understand if you've experienced it yourself. At the time, I thought about what had happened every day, from the moment I got up to the moment I fell asleep. And I'm afraid that hasn't changed. The memory and the feeling of what happened is always there.

When I went back for a second visit, I wanted to talk about it, but it was just too hard. I was bottling everything up, and when I tried to raise the subject, we both got so upset. It was thought by others that it might be best for me to stay away from Joe for a little while. Perhaps my being there was just too soon, and too upsetting for him, when he needed to concentrate on his recovery.

Mary (Joe's Mum):

It was bad at the time, but they're good now. The family pulled together, and I know that helped both of them, slowly, to accept what had happened, and start to move on.

Paul (Joe's Brother):

It's only recently that we've all been able to talk about what happened as a family. We hadn't really talked about it before that, and it was difficult. But we're a close family, We're there for each other. We didn't talk about specific things, but I think we all felt able to talk about the day and what had happened since. I still find it hard to accept, but Joe told me it wasn't my fault.

Joe:

Paul felt guilty and I know he still does. It was hard for me knowing what he must have been going through – and my whole family were going through – but even then, I knew that I had brought it on myself. If only, I had worn a seatbelt. But I was going to have to learn ways of dealing with the reality of what had happened to me if I was ever going to move towards a new life for myself.

I had always been a control freak, I liked things to be done my way or there'd be trouble! I had lived in a world where if I needed things to happen, I had been able to make them happen. The accident changed all of that. It restricted my ability to take control of situations, and that completely changed my outlook.

Sam (Joe's Sister):

It must have been so frustrating for Joe knowing that he'd been building the life he wanted, only to watch it fall apart. He'd done so much and acquired such a good reputation and he was proud of how far he'd come. But I do believe that what Joe had achieved in the past helped to keep him going. That strength pulled him on.

Kate (Joe's Friend):

Joe was always a really strong willed, opinionated person before his accident, perhaps he's become even more strong-willed since his accident. Perhaps some people would go the other way, but not Joe. Even as a young man of 16 or 17, he knew what he wanted.

Katie (Senior Case Manager):

> Everybody's recovery journey is different, of course. Many people have very bad experiences through their accidents and injuries. But I think that who a person is pre-morbidity – before the accident or injury – does shine through. So many people have told me about the trauma they have experienced, and I find it almost impossible to believe just how positive they still are. At this stage, I hadn't yet met Joe, but when I did, I saw that his pre-morbidity sense of strength and resilience shone through.

Joe:

> I knew I would need to dig deep into that same strength of character I'd shown in making my business dreams come true to help me. It took me a very long time. There were many hard times, and arguments along the way, and I lost relationships that were precious to me. But I slowly learned to work with people and manage people in a better way. I slowly learned to live a new life, and I learned to trust the many people who would help me on my way…

Andy (Mentor Support):

> I'd been aware of Joe for a little while before we actually met, but it wasn't until he got to Sheffield from Leeds that I was able to speak to him. He was in a challenging position at that time, he had been through an awful lot, and understandably, he was finding it hard to process all the different advice he was getting.
>
> I don't think he knew quite what to make of me in our first meeting. We got on well enough, we're of a similar age and we chatted away, we're both Yorkshire lads, so there were some things in common. After that, I went back to see him every fortnight when I was in the spinal unit. We spent time getting to know each other, and I saw his family a couple of times. I talked to them about how people of a similar level of injury to Joe had managed to get on with their lives, and I was able to signpost them to people and places to see what other people had achieved. So they went off and explored those things, then came back to me with more questions. It was an evolving process.
>
> As a Support Coordinator I work with everybody that's been affected by spinal cord injury, or damage to their spinal cord, whether through trauma, or through illness, disease, or condition. If somebody acquires damage to the spinal cord leading to neurological deficit, I am here to support them, their families, their carers, and the healthcare professionals who work with them. I provide peer support, drawing on my own lived experience. Sharing aspects of my own life can really help show somebody that life can go on after injury.

But it's important to appreciate that everyone's experience is entirely different, and my own experience as a low-level paraplegic might not initially seem that relevant to somebody like Joe. And when we first met, he was a little reluctant to engage with me. But as he found out, there is a lot of benefit in understanding my period of overcoming and adjusting to my own circumstances. But also, having been doing this job for so long now, I can draw on so many other examples of people of similar level injury or need.

It does obviously help that when I meet people with a spinal cord injury for the first time, they know that I've been there too. That's our icebreaker straightaway! It can help them feel a little bit more comfortable in talking about what they're going through and what they're dealing with, knowing that I've been through similar things. Never exactly the same things – everyone's experience is different – but similar.

Moving forward, when we've developed that understanding of each other, it makes it easier to talk. Not just about the injury and its effects, but about everything. Then, we're just two average people who have both faced an extraordinary situation.

I know from my own experience just how incredibly important that level of support is, not just from spinal cord injured people, but from many people who had had a lifelong or acquired disability. Just by seeing that I could do something, potentially they could – It's a powerful thing.

If you get in touch with us, or with anyone else who can support you in this way, you will be meeting with somebody who understands what you are going through. Having the confidence that the person you are talking to is considerate of what you're going through and has a strong understanding of it, and can therefore offer the kind of support and advice that is relative to your situation, as well as your friends, family and carers.

Joe:

I set up my charity, Quad-Rebuild, to help people who need support and practical help and advice. You'll find out more about at the end of this book.

5 On My Way Back

Eager to return to something approaching the life he knew, Joe threw himself back into work at the earliest opportunity, but was it too much, too soon?

The will is strong, what do I do with my life?

Joe:

By the time I was a bit more stable, a sense of determination to do something was growing in me. Even though, the anger was still there, and the physical limitations made it almost impossible, I felt the drive and determination to get back to work in some sense. The full reality of what life was going to look like hadn't fully sunk in yet, and I was keen to carry on with all of my construction work. At first everyone told me I had to let it go, but I suppose I was still in denial at the time.

I felt as if I could put a marker down that I was on my way back. So straight after they got me up in hospital, I felt ready to work. It was around three months after leaving intensive care. At first, my family and friends helped, (then later, I was able to use an eyegaze mouse stick system with a touchscreen computer and work more autonomously).

Ross (Joe's Friend):

Some of us felt as if he just needed to relax and get a bit further into his recovery and not bother about the business, but he really wanted to carry on. We'd seen him as close to death as its possible to be and then within a few weeks he was in his hospital bed quoting for jobs!

Peter (Joe's Dad):

Joe went back to his work very quickly. I thought it was too soon at first, but he had a big job on. Building work is stressful enough

DOI: 10.4324/9781003430728-6

as it is, and I didn't want him dealing with all of that stress on top of everything else. Most of all, he had the added stress of not being there. They had to send him photos and use FaceTime to show him what they were doing on the site.

Mary (Joe's Mum):

People rallied round and carried on the work for him, and he had drawings brought into him in Sheffield so he could price them. He couldn't stop thinking about it, he needed to focus on it so he could take his mind off other things.

Sam (Joe's Sister):

As soon as he was able to, Joe got to work from his hospital bed. We all worried that it was too soon, but we came to realise that he needed it. He coordinated with his team to complete that job. Everyone in the team pulled together and finished the job off to his satisfaction, and that helped him to carry on and focus on something more positive.

Ross (Joe's Friend):

In the end, we just had to stop worrying and help him. And I have to say that maybe Joe knew best all along, because within no time at all we were just talking and doing the work, and all the other pressures lifted off him. It was nice.

By the time he left Leeds for Sheffield, and we were able to see him more often, it did start to feel like it had before; we were just lads having a laugh. For that hour or so when we were there, it took him out of himself a little bit.

Joe:

I had unbelievable support and encouragement from my family and friends. They were with me every day, and that was massive for me. They used to bring architectural drawings and plans in for me to look at. Michelle brought her laptop so I could carry on talking to clients. When everything else was lost to me, I still had that. I'd had that desire in me since the first time I went out with my dad when I was just four or five years old, and it helped to keep me going. I wasn't going to let it go without a fight.

Barry (Joe's Friend):

When I asked him why he was carrying on with J. English Builders, he said he needed something to do. He said he could still do it, and his pride wouldn't let him hear anything to the contrary. Even then, in those very early days after his accident, you could see that he still had so much left to give.

Ross (Joe's Friend):

I know Joe likes to keep busy, and he always has. I think that had its difficulties during his recovery. After he threw himself back into it, he found it difficult to coordinate everything from afar. There were times when he felt as if some of the lads weren't doing the work they were supposed to be doing on site. He wasn't there to oversee it, and I think that was a massive frustration for him.

Joe:

I had always said to Michelle, "Work is always there for us, but people aren't." There were some people who took advantage of my not being there, and it made things increasingly difficult. The business had been going so well, but without me being there every day to look after things, it wasn't sustainable

Ross (Joe's Friend):

You'd take it for granted – just being able to go around and look at jobs, and see what everybody was doing, but he couldn't. Understandably, he fell out with a few people over that because they were letting him down. He felt they were taking the piss by not doing their best work for him, or leaving the site early. For someone like Joe, someone so hardworking and dedicated, it was really difficult for him to manage that. He was a man who would do it all himself if he could, and after the accident, he couldn't rely on other people to do it for him.

Sam (Joe's Sister):

Joe had never been comfortable relying on anyone else to do things he knew he could do himself. But being in hospital was a bit different. He knew he had to rely on his nurses and doctors. We knew the hospital staff were doing everything for him that they could, but they had other patients to see too, and I think his anxiety kicked in massively whenever we had to leave.

I never liked leaving him. But, particularly after he moved to Sheffield, those visits took up a big chunk of our time. We all had to go on working, and then we'd make the trip to see Joe. It took me an hour there to get there, and an hour to get back, and then off to work in the morning. It was like that for a whole year, and it was hard, but nothing was going to stop me seeing him. We've always been a close family, we've always been there for each other, no matter what, so nothing was going to stop us. We would have done anything Joe needed us to do for him.

But I would say that if you are in that position now, don't underestimate the toll it can take on you. Don't underestimate the pressure it can put on your day-to-day life. Give yourself as much time to look after yourself as you can. That's important for the person you're visiting, as much as for your own sake.

Prepare to be surprised too. Even after such a horrific accident tears through your family, you will find yourself smiling again. There will plenty of tears, but there will be laughter too. And all sorts for unexpected benefits...

Ross (Joe's Friend):

Seeing Joe go through all of this can't help but make you appreciate the little things all the more. My wife says I'm a different person because of it. After I come home from seeing Joe, I don't feel as if I can moan about the things that aren't quite right in my life. It has helped put everything in perspective.

I think we've all asked ourselves – if I were in Joe's position would I have wanted to carry on? Would I have been able to carry on? I still can't quite believe how Joe can be so positive about it. There have obviously been some times when he was really down, when everything just felt too painful for him. But he weathers every storm. And if you're in the position of worrying about a friend or loved one, I can tell you that there will be times where you have to do the hard work on behalf of your friend, but there will probably be times when they surprise you. That was certainly the case with Joe; there were times when I felt as if he was helping all of us get through it. And that's the mark of the man.

Katherine (Neuropsychologist):

In those early days of his recovery, Joe was starting to accept the position he was in, but only on the basis that he wanted to drive forwards and keep going. His return to work from his hospital bed gave him something new to focus on, but while Joe was showing laudable ambition and endeavour, I don't think that, at that stage, he was open to the concept of acceptance. A sense of urgency to drive forward and to prove something can be a bit of a sidestep.

Joe:

I didn't want to wait, I had things to do, and I wanted to get on with my life. But I knew there were certain things I couldn't control, which for me, was really difficult to deal with. And there was one thing in particular, that I was going to have to deal with that was going to take all of my strength to survive...

6   The Breakup

Not all of the effects of the crash were instantaneous, some of the aftershocks hit home much later. And when Joe's relationship unravelled, it threatened to plunge him back into depression.

No matter how much people love you, they can only be a punching bag for so long.

Mary (Joe's Mum):

> I spoke to Joe on the morning of the accident, and he wasn't his usual self. It was obvious that something was wrong, and he told me he'd had an argument with Michelle. Looking back, it's horrible to think that was the last conversation they had before the accident. I could tell he felt guilty about the argument. Joe was sure that Michelle was his soul mate, and it really hurt him when they argued.
>
> How must that have felt for her? In the morning they fought on the phone, and the next thing she knew, he was fighting for his life. After the accident, Joe wanted her with him, constantly. Michelle was a nice girl, and she was there for him when he really needed it, but of course she hadn't thought their lives were going to be like that…

Michaela (Joe's Sister):

> When Joe's life fell apart, it happened so suddenly. But the aftershocks took longer to play out. Without him there to look after it, the business started to struggle. The future that he'd been planning for slowly started unravelling. And then the cracks started to appear in his relationship with Michelle. She did stay with him for several months after the accident, but it was difficult. Joe was different…

Joe:

> I know I was too demanding with Michelle, just as I was too demanding of the staff at the hospital, and with my family. I couldn't

DOI: 10.4324/9781003430728-7

cope with losing control over any aspect of my life, let alone every aspect of my life. At the time, I couldn't understand why people didn't want to come and see me. Some of them said: if you don't get your own way you don't like it. Like they were speaking to a child. I couldn't make anyone understand how it felt: when you have been in control of your life, building your own destiny, and then have it all stripped away from you, that feels impossible to deal with. Then you add in the slow death of my relationship, and I felt lost.

Barry (Joe's Friend):

I know his relationship was a big worry for him. From the outside looking in, you see an attractive, young, able-bodied person in a relationship with a guy, who overnight, had been made quadriplegic, and who would need constant, round-the-clock care for the rest of his life. Coldly and objectively, it was obvious to me that she would want more from her life with a partner at that age. I think it would have been a different story if they'd been together for years, or if they'd both been a lot older, but their relationship was still young, and I knew that at some stage, Joe was going to have to consider letting her go.

It was hard for Joe of course, and in his own mind he wrote a different story at first. In the early days after the accident, he needed a dream of the future in which they were together, and they got a house, and they stayed together. He needed it to help pull him through some of his darkest days. He couldn't look beyond that.

Mary (Joe's Mum):

At first, she was planning ahead with him. She was saying, "We'll get you this, and we'll be able to go there…" They wanted to make it seem like everything could be like it had been before. But we could see it changing, and we knew that Michelle wasn't going to stay with him. Perhaps Joe knew it too, but he couldn't let himself believe it.

Joe:

It didn't happen all at once, but I could see the signs. At the start, I couldn't understand why she stopped coming to see me every day. I should have given her the space she needed. She'd sacrificed so much to be by my side for so long. But I think I was a bit selfish at the time.

She moved away to London, and at first, she came to see me every weekend, then every other weekend, then once a month, and then the excuses started. I couldn't control my anger then, and I knew, even then, that I wasn't projecting a very nice image of myself.

I kept asking her why she wasn't coming to see me, or where she was, which only pushed her further away. I was so wrapped up in my own little bubble. Now, I feel that if I'd eased off, things might have been different. But, of course, we'd both changed. I had changed beyond recognition, and she had been forced to change and adapt to that. In the end, I think I drove her away.

Mary (Joe's Mum):

In the end, he had to ask her to come and see him. He couldn't help it, he was still hanging onto the future they'd imagined. Most of all, he was so sad that he couldn't have a family of his own. He thought he'd never have a girlfriend again, he's said I can't even move my arms, I can't ever hug someone. But you never know. He's surprised us in so many ways.

Joe:

It still hurts. I loved her, and I know that she loved me. I didn't ever want to let her go. We were very passionate, very driven; very like-minded. She was my best friend; she was the person that I thought I would spend the rest of my life with. But I had to try and accept that the dream of our future was destroyed in the crash.

What do you do when something takes your whole future out from under you? I'd had dreams of us seeing the world. Our work would have taken us to London, Madrid, or Paris. We would have studied the architecture, done the work we loved doing, and then retire early and enjoy living our lives together.

But then everything that we had worked so hard for and everything we had accomplished was just taken away from us. It wasn't just what we'd lost. Our entire future went with it. And I was angry all over again.

From speaking to Katherine, my psychologist, since, I know that Michelle probably would have had a lot of anger about the accident too. It didn't just take her away from me; it had taken me away from her. And then there was all the abuse and trauma that followed.

By February 2020, I knew in my heart that she had moved on. I didn't know if I lost her because of the injury, or because of the anger that I projected towards her. And there were others. Friends who I pushed away. I felt the loss of it all over again. I had lost Michelle, I had lost my business, and I had lost my whole life. I can still feel the rawness of that separation, of everything that I had lost. I had survived so much, but I didn't know how to move on from Michelle. I didn't know if I could survive that. She's still in my mind now.

In the four years since the accident, she had been in my life for half of it. In the last few months, I have started to accept that she has moved on. I don't think there is any one thing I can recommend to you that will help, except to say, acceptance is key. Maybe my biggest problem, the reason I found acceptance hard to come by was because, I was – and am – such a control freak! But I know that if you don't accept what has happened to yourself, you will drive people away. No matter how much people love you, they can only be a punching bag for so long. Sooner or later, if you're not careful, the people who love you will drift away. You might never be able to move again, you might be paraplegic or have a head injury, but if you don't embrace what you have in the world, then the reality of what you don't have will eat you up, and it will destroy your relationships.

You've got two choices, it's that simple. You can give up, or you can face it head-on. Whether it's a relationship with a carer, a family member, or a friend, you have to remember that it's difficult for them too. That person or those people have no real way of knowing where you're coming from. They can't ever imagine what your life is like now, or what you're going through.

Michaela (Joe's Sister):

We're so grateful that Joe still has a life – and compared to some people – it's still a pretty good one, but we all know how much he suffered and how much he lost that day. We know there have been days when he's been close to feeling like giving up, when he's said, I can't do this anymore. Because we know that every day is a struggle for him in so many ways that the rest of us just haven't ever experienced and can't properly imagine. And the hardest part of all was knowing that he was there, on his own, crying in the dark, knowing he couldn't even wipe his own tears away.

Joe:

That's where I really hope this book will help. If you're like me, and you're coping with losing someone because of what has happened to you, I hope it will help you see that, even though it seems impossible, things do get better, I promise you. I couldn't imagine my life without Michelle, and there are still times when I find it hard to accept that she's gone. It didn't get better quickly, and as you'll read later, I was still dealing with it – consciously or unconsciously – when I started working with the neuropsychologist, Katherine Dawson. But here I am, writing about it now, and I'm doing alright. In many respects, I'm doing better than alright. As Michaela says, it's a pretty good life.

If you're reading this as a friend, a carer, or a loved one, I hope this book helps you to understand – even if it's just a little bit – that the person you care for is still in there. But they probably feel like they are going through hell, and for a while, it might feel like you've got no hope of reaching them. I am here to tell you that even if it feels like you're banging your head against a brick wall, you mustn't give up on them.

Andy (Mentor Support):

Joe is absolutely right. His story is a powerful reminder of what somebody can overcome. Think about the journey he has been on. When you consider his level of injury, it is astonishing that he kept on carrying on. But he did. In my work, I use Joe as a perfect example of just what somebody can achieve post-injury. Even in those early days of his recovery, and in spite of everything, we could sense his will to achieve something more with his life...

Part 2
It Takes a Village
The Team and the Technology
Supporting Joe's Recovery

7 "This Is What Your Life Is Going to Look Like…"

The transition from hospital to a specialist spinal unit was challenging on many levels. It brought home the reality of Joe's situation to him, leaving him in no doubt about his prospects.

I had been such an independent person before, and it was hard to let that go. I still didn't know how to let go.

Peter (Joe's Dad):

Even while Joe was still in Leeds, we started drawing up plans for an extension on my house. We knew he couldn't have gone back to his little town house. There were a few arguments along the way, and Joe will swear blind that it's all his work. He says. 'look at the value I've added to your house!' He's forgetting that I paid for it… and I lost my lawn!

But I knew he would need somewhere to come back to when he got out of hospital, where he could still be as independent as possible. We didn't want him going into a home. Funnily enough, he'd come over a few weeks before the accident, and talked to me about moving in for a bit. I said no!

Joe:

All of that was still a long way off. The next big step in my journey back home was getting out of Leeds and into a specialist spinal centre…

Rohit (Spinal Injuries Consultant):

Whenever somebody sustains a spinal cord injury in England or Wales, their information is uploaded on the national spinal cord injury database. Depending on which hospital the person is admitted to, the nearest designated spinal cord injury centre gets informed. Joe was admitted to Leeds Critical Care unit following his injury, and would ordinarily have gone to the Pinderfields Spinal Cord

DOI: 10.4324/9781003430728-9

Injury centre at Wakefield. However, given that he was on a ventilator, he was referred to the Sheffield spinal injuries centre as we are able to look after patients on a ventilator. At Sheffield, we get patients from South Yorkshire, the East Midlands, and the East of England regions.

People on ventilators are managed in an intensive care setting before they come to the spinal cord unit. This usually means that they are used to having one-to-one care at all times. There is always somebody around them, and this helps them to feel safe and supported. But in terms of their rehab and onward progress this can act as an impediment. It is important for us to empower our patients and try to reinforce a new sense of independence. One of the first things people notice after coming to the unit is that they won't have a nurse standing around, all the time, to help them. Initially, people may struggle to come to terms with that, but within the first few days they realise how that will help them once they get discharged from the hospital.

Joe was no different. He arrived around Christmastime, and I was on call when he arrived. He was obviously quite anxious to start with and worried how he would call for help if he needed it. It is our job to try and allay those fears and reassure our patients that they will always get the support they need, when they need it. I spoke to him at the time and was able to reassure him that this was the best next step in his rehab journey. You can't remain in the Intensive Trauma Unit for the rest of your life, and the centre is a kind of stepping-stone towards eventual discharge, whenever that happens down the line.

Joe:

I went from intensive care where I was used to one-to-one care, to a spinal injury unit, where it was one carer to every four people, and being in the unit was difficult. I remember the move very clearly. The thought of moving anywhere after so many weeks of being in the same place was scary, and they gave me a sedative to help me cope with the hour and a half hour journey. Shifting from the ventilator I'd been on in Intensive Care to a new ventilator was a traumatic process, and it took me a while to calm down enough to feel safe again.

Katherine (Neuropsychologist):

I hadn't met Joe at this point, but I can tell you that as an inpatient in a spinal cord injury unit, a person can experience a pronounced sense of loss and isolation. Initially there is, understandably, more of a focus on the physical aspects around managing pain, dealing with spasms, and bowel management. But, because of the enormity of what has happened, this phase of recovery is as much about helping somebody to understand and adjust. Psychology can be very useful in that sort of setting in just allowing people to be sad, and in identifying some of the common psychological consequences of a spinal cord injury. Often there is trauma involved because of the nature of the accident, so we may need to do some educative work around that.

At that early stage, people might not yet be connecting with the long-term implications of what has just happened to them, so part of what we do is to provide some psychological scaffolding for the future, which can cover mindfulness, relaxation techniques etc.

People have to adjust to new restrictions, to loss of independence, and emerging feelings around shame and vulnerability, and the grief around the loss of the lives they had imagined for themselves. Essentially the task is in helping someone to find a sense of hope, something to help them adjust to the change, and this can take a very long time.

Joe:

Those first six to eight weeks in specialist unit were very tough. I felt like nobody liked me. I know now that I was very aggressive and demanding. I had an attitude of 'I want what I want', and I hated being so dependent on anyone else. I had been such an independent person before, and it was hard to let that go. I still didn't know how to let go.

It wasn't a good start. It got to the point where nurses didn't want to come and help me. Rohit had a word with me and advised me that if I didn't calm down, they would have to move me to a different spinal centre. It wasn't just the staff I was upsetting, it was the other patients too.

Looking back, I feel that my inner control freak was in full flow, and I was still raging at being so powerless to help myself in any way. I know I was like a bull in a china shop, but the message got through, and I took a mental step back and reassessed my situation. And if you're in this situation, I can only recommend that you try and do the same. I know it's difficult, but if I had been a bit calmer and dealt with the situation in a more measured way, I could have moved through some of that anger more quickly. Instead of swearing my head off, I should have tried to articulate my concerns more calmly, and then I feel as if we could have addressed them, one by one.

Rohit (Spinal Injuries Consultant):

When the person has settled in and grown more used to their new routine, it's important that we talk to them about what has happened, and what is going to come next. Until that point, the critical care team will have focussed on telling their patients that they have had a spinal cord injury, and the details of any surgery they have had. Their focus is all about what is important here-and-now. Our role at the Spinal Injuries centre is to move that conversation from the 'present' to the 'future'. We need to address candidly what the injury means in real terms. About what impact it will have on their body over the next few months and years. We talk about impairments to bladder and bowel function, and other organ systems that may be affected from their injury. And we talk about what they can expect in the short- and long-term.

These are obviously difficult conversations to have, but in any specialist unit like ours, there is a lot of expertise available. There are people who can direct those kinds of conversations in the right way. The doctors, consultants and specialist nurses are all trained to look after spinal cord injury patients. Our physiotherapists and occupational therapists (OTs) are specialists in spinal cord injury rehab.

For patients, the learning is often incremental: when the physio sees the patient to run through physio routines, when the OT sees them to discuss hand functions, and when the specialist nurse sees them for bowel care, it all helps develop the patient's awareness of what is happening to them. Every healthcare professional involved understands what spinal cord injury is, and every one of those small interactions with the patient contributes to further understanding, and ultimately, acceptance.

If I were to go and see a new patient on their first day and tell them, "This is what your life is going to look like..." it wouldn't be a very helpful kind of induction. But if instead, a new patient interacts with the whole specialist team over the course of a couple of weeks, they start to realise the full extent of their injury. They come to appreciate what they need, and why they need it, and that gradual understanding eventually leads on to a one- or two-hour meeting with the consultant a month or two down the line to discuss the injury and its consequences in more detail. This is when we show the person their scans, if they want to see them, so they can see what a spinal cord injury actually looks like. They'll see what the injury has done to their spine and spinal cord, which can help them form a greater appreciation of their new limitations.

Joe:

I remember this conversation very well. There was a room with a big television on the wall where they showed me the break in my spinal cord. I had some of my family with me, and as I looked at the pictures, I felt numb. The reality of my situation had been growing more and more clear, but that was the moment when it became official; I was never going to improve.

Rohit carried out a pinprick test, gently touching the surface of my skin to demonstrate the loss of feeling all over my body. It was dawning on my family too. Any dreams they might have had that I would suddenly get better ended that day.

As a control freak, I had never liked being told by people what my future was going to look like. I felt as if they didn't have the right to limit my future like that. I wanted to know what all my options were, and my family did too.

Andy (Mentor Support):

I know that when families leave their loved ones in the hospital after an event like this, many of them will be tempted to go and research things online. Unfortunately, there is a lot of unhelpful or inaccurate information out there. Start with trusted resources like the Spinal Injuries Association website and Quad-Rebuild; they are both great sources of support and advice, and they are checked regularly to ensure that it is absolutely up-to-date.

Michaela (Joe's Sister):

I didn't want to believe it. When the doctors in ITU had told us what Joe would or wouldn't be able to do, I wanted to see for myself what other people had experienced. I ended up doing a lot of Googling; I wanted to try and find out if there was anything we could do to help Joe. But that day in the spinal injury unit, everything changed.

Rohit (Spinal Injuries Consultant):

I appreciate that Joe and his family felt as if his hopes and expectations were crushed when he was in ITU. And it is only natural for patients and their families to want to look for stories of people who have overcome all the odds to recover.

That's why seeing the injury is a very important part of the process for many people. Having a visual understanding of what has happened helps them make those connections… my bladder isn't working, my hand isn't moving – now I can see and understand why. Typically, by the time a person has the meeting with the consultant a month or two down the line, patients will have developed a very good understanding of the situation. They will know from the work they have been doing, and the limitations they have been working around, just how severe the spinal cord injury is, and what it means for them, both now and in the longer term. So, this is the point at which we'll start to talk more seriously about what might be achievable, and what we would expect them to do in the future.

One of the frequent questions I get asked by patients when presented with what their new circumstances might look like is: 'How do you know?' My usual answer is that we are making these predictions based on our clinical examination and findings. These give us a very reliable sense of how a person's injury is going to evolve or progress. Most patients follow this trajectory of neuro-recovery. There are always exceptions, and some people get more recovery than others.

Through our examination, we try and get answers for two important questions:

What is the level of injury?
What is the severity of injury?

The spinal cord runs from the base of the brain all the way down to the tail bone. You can have an injury at the neck level, or at the upper back level, or the lower back level. This will help determine the neurological level of a person's paralysis. In Joe's case, the injury was just below where the base of the brain and the spinal cord meets, it's called the C3/C4 region. That is high enough to affect the phrenic nerve which supports our breathing. That's why Joe ended up needing a ventilator to breathe.

The severity of injury tells us how severe or dense the injury is. It can vary from being quite severe (complete paralysis below the level of injury) to being extremely mild (getting near-complete recovery). We label these severities from A (dense) to E (full recovery).

Based on our assessments, Joe had severe spinal cord injury at the neck resulting in complete paralysis from the neck down.

Most online success stories do not reveal the full details of a person's injury severity. Of course, there are stories about people who have had seemingly remarkable recoveries after a spinal injury.

The level of the injury is important, but we are also looking at the severity of the injury. On one end of the spectrum, you can get an injury which leaves a very small scar on the spinal cord, while the rest of the spinal cord continues to function. That person will experience very minimal deficits as a result of their injury.

Andy (Mentor Support):

I was relatively lucky. I couldn't ever have imagined it in my darkest days, but I did achieve a significant level of recovery. There is still a significant deficit, and I'll always be a wheelchair user, but I was able to effectively start a new life. Now I have a wife and two daughters, I work four days a week, nine-to-five, I drive, I go on holiday, I drop the kids off at school; I really live a very average life!

Of course, I did still have to make that adjustment to a new normal, and it did take time. The nature of Joe's injury meant that his outlook was somewhat different.

Rohit (Spinal Injuries Consultant):

Unfortunately, Joe sustained a very dense injury. The research and case studies show that if you start off with a less dense injury, the chances of improvement are much greater. But sadly, the more severe the injury is, the smaller the chances of making a full recovery.

The conversations we have on the ward slowly start to suggest this to the patient; our job then is to work towards helping the patient to come to terms with the reality of it through all those little conversations and interactions. It means we can start to talk about living life in a wheelchair, and discuss how one might be able to manage that. We talk about what leisure activities one enjoyed before, and what might still be possible after the accident or injury.

Joe:

It is one of the most important lessons you'll learn: our recoveries are all going to be different. It's not just our injuries that are different, it's who we are as people to begin with. People will tell you that I was always very driven and that helped me to stay focussed on doing anything I could to improve after the accident.

Katie (Case Manager):

I hadn't met Joe at this point, but he raises a really important point. Whoever a person is before the accident – their pre-morbid condition – is a good indicator of the sort of response they might have to the recovery process, and it can help people better understand the kind of support they'll need.

Obviously, I don't have the privilege of meeting anyone before their injury, but when I speak to family and friends, I will ask if they have noticed any differences in the patient's memory or behaviour. You can expect behaviours to change in the immediate aftermath when patients may be overwhelmed by what has happened to them. Very often people will say to me, "Oh, she was always like this! Always a bit bad-tempered!" In general, people don't undergo a personality transformation. Even if there is a hint of that temporarily, the pre-morbid personality usually shines through in the end. And when I met Joe later, I soon discovered that he had always been a very driven, very positive person pre-morbidity.

But of course, we are not all positive people. And I think it is important for friends and family to be aware that if the patient has always been more of a glass-half-empty person, then they might need that bit more support to stay positive.

Rohit (Spinal Injuries Consultant):

Just as everyone else has said, my first impression of Joe was that he was a very driven person. He was running his own business from a young age. He had achieved so much through hard work and focus, so he inevitably found it difficult to accept that he wasn't going to have that same level of control over his day-to-day situation any more. Over the course of those first few weeks, it must have felt as if a lot of professionals were telling him what to do, and I know he found that challenging.

As professionals, we understand what our patients are going through, and we are only ever there to help them. But we also know how difficult the situation can seem to our patients. There were times when Joe may have said something to me in the heat of the moment, but I would never have any reason to take that personally. I knew it was just an expression of his frustration borne of what was happening.

Even with such a high-level injury, Joe's drive and determination inspired him to take back control of as many aspects of his life as he could, and he was soon back to managing aspects of his business by phone. In all my time working with ventilated patients, I'd never seen anyone else do that. Once Joe started doing that, he found new purpose and something to focus on which made his situation easier to manage. After that, it was much easier to talk to him about rehab because he started to take on board the things that he would need to return to his life.

Joe was well on his way to becoming an expert patient. But unfortunately, not everyone gets the same level of care post-ITU.

Andy (Mentor Support):

Sadly, there are a lot of people with spinal cord injuries, or damage to the spinal cord who don't get treated in a spinal unit because they don't meet the NHS criteria for admission. Very often this will be because of the presence of cancer; the spinal injury services are unable to support cancer care, and the cancer care will always take priority. Before the nurse specialist services provision was in place, we were seeing too many people sadly dying from relatively minor spinal cord complications like a pressure sore, or poor continence leading to sepsis, even though their cancer prognosis gave them a relatively good life expectancy. Hence the need for the clinical nurse service to support spinal cord injured people and their carers, ensuring that their needs are being met, whether that's in an acute hospital, a rehab centre, or at home, post-discharge. I was lucky enough to get a huge amount of support and education from the spinal injury services, so was Joe. That's why it's so sad to see people missing out if they don't go on that same pathway.

But now with our own SIA, and Joe's Quad-Rebuild charity, there are options for everyone reading this book, whatever your situation. I know that support from the Spinal Injuries Association really can be a life saver for people. We offer specific peer-led counselling that really is worth its weight in gold. Spinal cord injured people and their friends and families don't have to go through the arduous process of explaining the implications of the injury to a counsellor before actually getting to talk about whatever they need to talk about. Their counsellor will already be well aware of the implications of the injury.

We have an advocacy service, so we can advocate for anyone who needs a voice. We make sure their needs are heard, and we'll help get them what they need. I will often speak on behalf of people to get their housing issues dealt with, to get their equipment requests sorted, and beyond that, I can advocate for care funding. Continuing healthcare funding (CHC) is a big aspect of our work. It's that kind of funding that pays for the ongoing care of people, like Joe, who really need it. Generally, higher-level care people who need funding will get CHC. We can help a person get their care plan in place if they're not going through a spinal unit, and put a proposal to the CHC team to ensure they get the right amount of funding for their care needs. Then, when people are in the community, their care packages will undergo continual review, and may be reduced. Anyone who is early on in their recovery may struggle to know how to tackle that, so we can be there to support them.

The Spinal Injuries Association and the support network which is now in place has many other beneficial services, including a nurse specialist service, focussing on people that are not being treated by a spinal specialist rehabilitation centre. We can link up with other services, whether they're in-house or external services that will be useful in helping them move forwards in life as soon as possible. This network includes other charities, including benefits advice, wheelchair skills, community engagement, equipment provision, housing, holidays, care partners and care providers, financial advisors, legal teams and more. It's a constantly evolving network to help meet the needs of a disparate group of people as they move on in life after injury, and its constantly reviewed to identify any trends so we can look at partnering with providers in those areas or develop our own in-house provision.

Joe:

The question that hung over me was: *How am I going to live my life now?*

Seeing what sort of help was available for people like me – and more importantly, what sort of help wasn't available – stirred something in me. The feeling that I didn't just want to lie there and take it. I needed to get better so I could do something important with my life while I was growing stronger...

8   What Can You Expect in Rehab?

It isn't just physical rehabilitation, an effective rehab process takes a more all-encompassing view of a patient's needs after a life-changing injury, enabling them to move forwards more confidently.

This is effectively where I was reborn... they teach you how to live the rest of your life.

Rohit (Spinal Injuries Consultant):

If you or a loved one is preparing to enter rehab, what can you expect?

Many people's expectations of rehabilitation focusses on what happens in the therapy hall with the physios, or in the gym or occupational therapy unit. And we know that the more time people spend in bed rest, the more they get deconditioned, so the approach we take on a rehab ward is to try and get people moving as quickly as possible.

Some of the most significant improvements a person can make are functional improvements, e.g. getting a movement back that enables one to carry out a certain action. Joe did have some minor sensory improvements, but no functional improvements.

But of course, this process isn't just about physical rehabilitation. For our patients, rehab revolves around a core of dedicated physiotherapy sessions, dedicated occupational therapy sessions, and psychology support.

We understand that this is a life-changing injury that no one has prepared for. Suddenly you are expected to be able to deal with all of the problems and challenges that come with it. A spinal cord injury affects almost every organ system in the body. It affects the way your bladder and kidneys work. It affects your bowel function; it even affects the way you sweat. It can affect respiratory function – as in Joe's injury – and that in turn can affect the way your heart works. In a specialist centre like ours, our aim is to help patients

DOI: 10.4324/9781003430728-10

achieve the best possible rehab outcome. That means providing a good understanding of what has happened to every patient, and working to maximise the abilities of every patient following injury.

So, a big part of the rehab process is to help you start to think about the life changes that are going to affect you, and very practically, what can be done to help you. Will you be able to go back to your home? If so, what modifications will you need at home? What support is available in the community to help you? These may be some difficult conversations to have, so we will approach them gradually, bit by bit, giving you time to adjust to your new circumstances.

As far as we are concerned, every conversation, every interaction with a specialist nurse or practitioner, and every new insight into their injury are equally important parts of the rehabilitation process. As I mentioned in the previous chapter, they all combine to start painting a picture of a new future for our patients.

We want to help our patients maximise their ability, and give them as much physical independence as possible. By the end of our work together, we want them to become expert patients. In other words, they should leave our care with enough insight and understanding of their spinal cord injury as possible, much more understanding than an average health professional in the community will have. And, if they are going to need carers, they need to be in a position to tell the carer – who may not have anything like the same understanding about spinal cord injuries – what is right or isn't right for their care. Education really is of paramount importance.

We will look at what you can expect, both in the near future, and in the long term. As a part of this ethos, anybody who is referred to us is given life-long follow-ups as and when they need them. Even after patients are discharged, we see them at three-months, six-months and one year after discharge. After that, we go on seeing them every year, and patients know they can contact us at any time if there is a problem.

It's important that by the time they leave, our patients don't feel cut off; we're always here if they need us. After everything that Joe has dealt with, he knows that he can still look to us for help. He has the contact numbers of our outpatient nursing teams, and whenever he needs us, he calls.

Joe:

Not everyone will know how to articulate what they want and need when they come out of hospital. My advice to people if they struggle a little bit is to take direction from people who have experienced what you have experienced – or something similar – and to use your time in hospital well.

Andy (Mentor Support):

There's no time limit on the sort of support you might need when you've had a spinal cord injury, it's a lifelong service. Once they're being supported by us, people can access our help and support whenever they want, for whatever reason. Some people – like Joe – are very proactive about getting in touch, so we have to be mindful of people who don't get in touch so readily, just to make sure that they're getting on alright.

Rohit (Spinal Injuries Consultant):

It is important to have that kind of reassurance, of knowing that you can refer to somebody who knows you and understands what you are going through. Whatever issues he may have, we will address them for him.

Having said that, our job is to prepare our patients for life outside the unit, so we are very much focussed on giving our patients everything they need to live as autonomously as possible. Clearly, this is a difficult road, but I always tell my patients that, while nobody plans for injuries like these, they can still make the best of their situation. And if you are in a situation where rehab is available to you, I strongly urge you to take any opportunity, whether that is through the NHS, or privately.

One of the guiding principles of our service is that the patient remains at the centre of everything that happens. We are here to support and help people whatever they want to achieve, based on their goals.

A spinal cord injury is life changing, but patients retain good thinking abilities and brain function; even if they are physically limited, patients can, in most cases and to varying degrees, still continue to engage in much of the same work and in leisure activities as they did before. I know of people who, after their spinal cord injury have returned (with suitable adaptations) to embrace their passion for sailing. I know of people who have taken up sports like wheelchair basketball and rugby. In fact, the vice captain of the GB Wheelchair Rugby Team which won gold at the Tokyo Paralympics, is one of our patients. There are still so many opportunities out there. Whatever a patient wants to do can normally be done, just in a slightly different way. Everybody takes that on board.

I appreciate there may be things which one is used to doing which may no longer be possible. In Joe's case, there was stone carving, which he simply cannot do in any adapted way. People tend to find that something else takes over; some other sporting or leisure activity that distracts them from what they can't do. Finding alternatives to those things makes a difference, or even trying something that you have never previously tried; something which can become a new passion. To help with that process, we have an Activities Coordinator in our unit, and she helps people to find alternative interests and engage people with different activities.

One of the main worries that patients have is the question of how other people will perceive them. I think that getting over that misgiving really helps people to move on. In my experience, other people understand that injuries like this are a regrettable part of life; there is no stigma, only support for these people. We do see excellent outcomes for patients who have had wonderful support from their families and friends.

Families do tend to get forgotten in all of this. But of course, they all have to experience their own journey in dealing with the impact on their lives. It's important that while they support their friend or loved one they remain well looked after too.

Michaela (Joe's Sister):

But don't forget your own needs. Reach out to people to get the help and support you need too. I'm lucky, I have a family around me who know exactly what I'm going through. I urge you to find someone you can talk to.

Rohit (Spinal Injuries Consultant):

It isn't always a good idea to take on roles and responsibilities that might take away their freedom. We know that a patient may require a significant level of care or support when they get discharged, but we don't often recommend that a spouse or family member takes up the job of caring for their loved one. We want to allow the dynamics between couples and family members to remain intact.

It is of course very helpful for spouses, family members and friends to learn the essential care techniques. That can make it easier for people to go on holiday after an injury without needing to engage as many carers in their holiday destination. Or, if there is an emergency, it is reassuring for everyone to know that the family member or friend can help straightaway.

During the time when patients are with us – which was 11 months in Joe's case – there are many opportunities for family and friends to come in and meet with us, and I recommend you do that. It allows us to involve them in parts of the process. We encourage spouses and family members to join us for that initial meeting with the patient; it's a good forum for them to ask questions. Very often, people coming in will ask extremely relevant questions about discharge and next steps. We can reassure them about the procedures we'll take, and the steps we'll put in place to make that transition as smooth as possible. All we really want is for them to be there to support our patient in an effort to try and get them back to a new normal as quickly as possible.

Joe certainly had his fair share of challenges, and at first, he found it difficult to deal with what had happened, in terms of the limitations that his injury placed on him. He found it difficult to interpret all those changes that his body was undergoing. He did have additional complications like chest infections, problems with his ventilator, and abdominal and bowel issues, none of which were unexpected given the severity of his injury. It took him some weeks to really come to terms with it all.

I'm jumping ahead a little bit here, but by the time Joe left us, he was an expert patient. He knew what his needs were, and he knew how to manage his situation. That, to me, feels like the best possible outcome.

Joe:

This is effectively where I was reborn. From a medical perspective, they teach you how to live the rest of your life. They will tell you how to look after your specialist clinical needs and how you should expect care agencies and carers to provide that care. That is vitally important for you in the build-up to your release from hospital. Lots of people that you'll meet outside of hospital may be experts in general medicine but won't necessarily be best placed to talk to you about issues relating to your situation.

When I didn't know what I know now, one of the nurses who had worked for a care agency talked to me about my flip flow valve. Normally when most people have a bladder full of urine, you hold onto it until their brain tells them that they need to release it. Following my injury, I had a little valve put in that flips down and releases the urine. When the catheter got blocked and I rang an ambulance, they had no clue about what a suprapubic catheter was, and disregarded my call as a non-emergency. I had to ring my district nurses to come and change the catheter. Many medical staff know very little about bladder and bowel management.

Everything that I was taught in hospital relating to medication, turning regime, how to look after my skin, my bowel and bladder routine, all of it stuck with me. It's so important that each individual follows the things that they have been taught that relate specifically to them and their condition.

9 Working with Your Case Manager

Your Case Manager will play a pivotal role in your process through rehabilitation and on into a new life. Here, you can find out what the role encompasses, and how to make the most of your relationship with your Case Manager.

I know that there is always something I can do to make a difference... whatever it might be that will help our client start to experience life a little more positively.

Katie (Senior Case Manager):

I will be instructed by a solicitor or an insurance company to provide case management for people going through litigation. That could be as a result of an accident, or clinical negligence, for example. Case managers may specialise in different disciplines, but we mainly focus on spinal cord injuries, as well as some clients with brain injuries, and some orthopaedic work.

We are drawn from related disciplines, so there are nurses, OTs, physios, and social workers; my own background is in occupational therapy. It's important to have a good level of clinical knowledge within that speciality.

I worked as an OT in the spinal unit in Sheffield for a number of years, and then I worked as a care service manager for a live-in specialist care agency for people with spinal injury and complex neuro disability, and that experience certainly helps me to manage expectations.

We can be instructed by the claimant's solicitor under single instruction, but in some situations it could be a joint instruction. In these cases, the claimant's solicitor would be working in a collaborative way with the defendant's solicitors who are representing the insurance company.

The clients I work with will have suffered a traumatic experience, or suffered from clinical negligence, for example if somebody went into hospital expecting that their back problem would be improved and came out of their surgery paralysed.

DOI: 10.4324/9781003430728-11

The work that we do will be partly dependant on what funds are available. In some cases, a client will have been given a lump sum of money, known as interim funds, intended for therapy, rehab work, appropriate equipment, things that may not be available from statutory services, or equipment that might be more specialised. Take wheelchairs as an example. We would assess a client who needs a wheelchair, and present them with the best option that their resources allow. But if there is additional funding, or private funding, we may be able to suggest something more ideal, with more appropriate seating, or one that we think will be easier for the client to use. It may be that a chair from wheelchair services will be appropriate, but any additional funding just allows us to explore more options on the client's behalf.

As a clinician you formulate ideas about what people might be able to achieve, and we look at a wide range of services and care provisions for our clients, and involve people who can help. Everything we do is client-centred. So we ask questions like these to ensure every client is receiving the best possible range of services and care:

Is their care appropriate?
Do we need to get involved in making sure they are getting the kind of care they need?
Do they need any additions to existing services?
Is their property suitable?

Perhaps I will assess someone and see that they don't have appropriate provision for neuro-physio, which could potentially really help them. Or I might find out that they really need some additional psychological support. Or there may be physical issues; perhaps they're living in a house that requires them to get mobile ramps out every day just to get in and out of the house.

Mary (Joe's Mum):

The practicalities are really important to help Joe live a full life. Like Katie said, if simple things like getting in and out of the house are too awkward, it can make life very difficult. Joe can't easily go to everybody's house because there isn't always wheelchair access.

Katie (Senior Case Manager):

I will identify what clients need, how much that is going to cost, what I can access from statutory services, and what will need to be privately funded, and I will put that to the client and whoever is instructing me. A decision will then be made, either to approve funds for those things or if there is an interim payment, the client can decide what they are going to spend their money on, and what they will prioritise. I have to support decisions that are reasonable and justified, but ultimately, it is for the client.

Joe:

Personal autonomy is really important. In the early days after my accident, I had no personal space, and no autonomy. I couldn't even remove myself from an argument, or a stressful situation. I couldn't get up and walk out of the room if I needed some space. Your home needs to feel like your safe space, and if there is funding available to help make that a reality, talk to your case manager to see what they can do to help you.

And if there is help and support you need beyond that, contact my charity, Quad-Rebuild. One of our missions is to help people find ways to modify their houses to accommodate their new circumstances.

Katie (Senior Case Manager):

The privilege that I have as a case manager is that I get involved because there is some degree of interim funding or private funding, and I know that there is always something I can do to make a difference. Whether that is getting more intensive physio, or more psychological support, or whatever it might be that will really help our client start to experience life a little more positively, we can put things in place they might not have experienced before. That doesn't necessarily mean better quality service provision than they may have had before, but it does almost certainly mean something that is more specifically focussed on them and their particular needs.

I can think of every one of my clients and know that I have been able to bring positive change and support. Very often, after discharge from hospital, things can feel very difficult. They may have limited access in their house, they may have a care agency that they regard as merely okay, and what they really need is someone who can bring all the elements together. If somebody has a care package that they're not happy with, they might struggle to get through to the care agency and articulate the issues. It may be that their needs have been miscommunicated, or that they are not getting the kind of support they really need. So, they can talk to me about those things, and I can take that burden off their shoulders and make some of those changes happen. Day to day can be enough of a struggle, so the more we can do to improve things on their behalf, the better.

Joe:

It's helpful to involve your family and friends in some of your discussions – but not all of them! Sometimes a committee is good, but other times your wishes trump all others, and that's how it has to be.

Katie (Senior Case Manager):

We do of course respect our clients' wishes as to how much involvement their family should have in the process, and indeed there might be some consent issues involved. Some clients will not want their families to get involved, for a wide variety of reasons, which we will respect absolutely.

Of course, the impact on our clients is the most significant, but it is also true that the accident or injury will have an effect on your nearest and dearest too. Family members will be facing their own journeys through recovery. We can work with family members too, if required, to offer appropriate support and counselling, or family therapy.

In many initial meetings, the client will be accompanied by a family member, and so I will always say that if there are any questions that either of them don't feel comfortable answering in front of each other, for any reason, then we will work around that. And then when I have time alone with the client, I will find out if there is anything that they wouldn't want talked about in a family situation. It's important we understand what the boundaries are.

Joe:

One of the reasons for writing this book is to help you get the best out of everyone who is there to help you. It took me a while to move from being very hands-on and very independent to allowing others in to help me.

Katie (Senior Case Manager):

If you are in the early stages of preparing to meet a case manager, this is how the process works.

Sometimes, I will get involved in a case because the solicitors or the insurers will have worked with me before, or I will have been recommended to them. But it's important to say: You get a say in this process too! You are at liberty to meet a number of case managers to help you decide who you want to work with.

Your solicitor or your insurance company will usually be able to source a case manager with the right clinical expertise, whether that is experience of orthopaedic injuries, spinal or brain injuries, working with amputees etc. Case managers have a lot of transferable skills, but it's certainly good to look at your prospective case manager's CV to learn more about their background and clinical experience.

Once you've agreed to start working with a case manager, they will assess your situation and make recommendations based on that assessment. Their recommendations can be wide-ranging, relating to clinical issues, support issues, or advice and support around leisure activities.

You will work together collaboratively. They will work with you and in your best interests at all times to source the right equipment, the right care, and the right services for you, and go on reviewing and overseeing everything. It's a responsive relationship too. For example, for clients who are parents, we would help to source the right kind of childcare, and facilitating their parenting following an incapacitating injury. We are there for the clients in difficult times. Clients need to know they can rely on their case manager; they will become a key part of the client's team.

I was asked to go and meet Joe for an initial chat, so we could get to know each other, and I think this is a really important part of the process. It means that you are able to quiz a potential case manager on their knowledge and experience and get a feeling for how they work.

Every case is different. In some cases, it is necessary to assess everything in great detail, in Joe's case we looked at the key, standout things that he wanted to address. It was 18 months after his accident when I met him. Joe was an impressive chap. At that time, he was still living in a small extension off his father's house. He was very positive, but also quite insightful with regard to his vulnerabilities and the position he found himself in. He already had lot of ideas about the future, and how he was going to continue his business, and set up a charity to help people whose lives had been affected like his.

Joe is a problem-solver. If he sees a potential barrier to something, he will find out how to get around it. He will sometimes tell me something that he wants to achieve, and as a case manager, I have to work with him to plot the steps to allow him to try and reach his end goal. I'm there to support my clients and work in their best interests, but equally I must be able to justify what I have recommended, and why I have or haven't done certain things.

If a client wanted to do something that I thought might be a bit risky, I wouldn't be doing my job properly if I didn't help them see the alternative options at their disposal to mitigate any risk.

Barry (Joe's Friend):

Joe being Joe, it didn't take long before he wanted to go on holiday, and he asked me if I'd go to Barcelona with him. After discussing it with his case manager and the carers, we realised he would need a specially adapted bed, we would have needed to have been close to a hospital, and if anything had happened, I didn't feel as if we'd have known what to do. I persuaded him instead that we should have some time in England – it was having quality time together that mattered after all.

Katie (Senior Case Manager):

I have a clinical responsibility and a duty of care, while also trying to help them strive to achieve more. I do sometimes have to be the person that says, "Just slow down a bit, we need to tick these boxes first." Ultimately, a client can do whatever they want to, whether I agree with it or not, but at the very least I need to make sure they have all the information at their disposal before they make their decision.

Of course, we will go on assessing and reassessing your needs and your capacity to do new things. What may not be possible or practical now, may be achievable in a few months or years' time. I will go on reviewing what progress is being made and assess whether the input of a physio or a psychologist should increase, decrease or stay consistent. We will also look to see if any elements of what is being provided can be handed over to carers. If progress isn't being made, it doesn't mean that that we took the wrong course or made the wrong decision, it might be that they're not ready for that kind of intervention. To give you a general example, psycho-sexual therapy is a good example of that. There are so many elements involved in that kind of work that although clients are keen to pursue it, they find that the timing just isn't right. When somebody has had a profound physical injury, they may find that there are other physical issues to address. Perhaps they are also experiencing issues with bladder and bowel care, for example, so the last thing they want to be talking about is sexual relationships.

That's why it's important to review progress on a regular basis to ensure we're achieving what we want – and what we expect – to achieve. If not, why not, and what can we do about that? We review what the client experience is like and see if they're happy with how things are progressing. Are the services being provided meeting their expectations?

It's important for us to have multi-disciplinary team meetings that bring together all the people working with the client, which could involve psychologists, physiotherapists, occupational therapists, and dieticians; this helps everyone to understand what is going on and what factors might impact on their own service provision.

In a case like Joe's, progress can be slow, just because of the nature of a spinal cord injury. I would request a report from the physio every 12 weeks which summarises their goals, and progress, with the specific things they are working on. They would also outline costs.

If a physio is working with a client for three months, and we're approaching the end of the three months then we would use that opportunity to review what we have achieved and what we haven't achieved – and why – so that we can set new goals for the following weeks, and what the estimated costs would be. This information goes to the client and whoever is funding them to ensure they're aware of our planned next steps. It's a fluid process, things don't tend to just stop.

I can be with a client from the litigation process through to settlement, and potentially beyond. Typically, there will be a provision within the settlement that they will continue to require case management for the rest of their lives.

In some cases, clients may decide that they want to become the employer of their own care team, rather than using a care agency, and in those cases, the case management input will usually be higher. The case manager will go on assisting and overseeing the process, on a lifelong basis. I have a couple of clients who have been settled a number of years who now employ their own care teams, and I am still involved to help, particularly with elements like recruitment and training.

If somebody in Joe's position decides that, in the long term, they would like to recruit their own staff, I would need to manage the clinical input, the resources for training, managing rotas, payroll, etc. In other words, case managing ranges from quite a light touch intervention to something much more involved.

Most of our clients do continue with some form of case management. It can also encompass things like support for a client who is going on holiday abroad for the first times in many years, and may require some assistance with that. Or people may go on to get married and may require some support with accessing a fertility clinic.

Of course, some people are able to become really independent like Joe, they don't need much input after a certain point and go on to do really well, with minimal support.

10   Rebuilding Your Life

Learning to see yourself for who you are – wheelchair and all – when you're used to thinking of yourself as an able-bodied person is one of the most challenging things you will ever have to do.

I had almost stopped thinking about myself as a physical being in a way... I wasn't ready to see myself in the wheelchair, and I wasn't prepared to come to terms with the fact I couldn't get out of the chair and walk.

Joe:

How do you look in a wheelchair?

I went a good six months before I was able to look at myself in the mirror. I came out of intensive care and into a rehab unit. I was lying in a bed for four-to-six-weeks. First, they just had to fight to keep me alive, then they had to try and regulate my bladder and bowel function, and feed me up a little bit. In ICU, I went down from 11-stone to just eight-stone.

When I got to rehab, I didn't even think about my appearance. That might sound strange; we're all used to looking at ourselves and checking our image, but when you've been though a profoundly life-changing experience, it alters everything. It took me so long to come to terms with being paralysed from the neck down that nothing else really registered. I wasn't thinking about looking in the mirror to see if I needed a shave or a haircut, or to check what I was wearing; I was focussed on my new situation.

As part of focussing on my new normal, I had to get used to all the new things that could go wrong. I was told that I might get dizzy – that's hypertension – if my blood pressure dropped below 50, and if that happened, I would pass out. Or at the other extreme, my BP could go sky high to 220 – that's autonomic dysreflexia – which can happen as a result of a bladder or bowel blockage which can be fatal if not treated properly.

DOI: 10.4324/9781003430728-12

Even now that I understand what can go wrong as well as anyone, things do still go wrong. And even though I eventually left the unit as an expert – as Rohit mentioned – it didn't mean that I could prevent some of those clinical emergencies from happening.

Mary (Joe's Mum):

As a parent or loved one, one of the hardest things to deal with is wondering if – or when – something is going to go wrong. Wondering when the boot is going to fall; he's had to go back to hospital a few times. Last time he was in hospital, he had to be put into a coma again.

Joe:

Jumping ahead in my story, I can tell you that I have had several further hospital admissions for some pretty serious issues...

One of the hardest things about having a spinal injury is that you cannot feel below your neck. Or, rather, they told me I would never have any feeling at all. Actually, I can feel touch down to the middle of my chest, but I can only feel pain from my neck upwards. It's not quite pain really, more the touch or the sensation of it without the actual pain.

Practically this means that I can't tell if my skin is burning in the sun, and I can't even tell if I've had too much to eat or drink. Most people know when it's time to stop eating because they begin to feel full, but what happens when you don't get those signals from your stomach? I love my food so it is particularly hard for me to decline food when my body can't tell me that I've had enough. I know that if I'm not extremely careful, I am at risk of my bowels blocking from eating too much; this causes dysreflexia which is extremely uncomfortable and potentially very dangerous.

In 2019, my bowels blocked and I ended up in hospital for over six weeks, nil by mouth. It happened again a year or two later. I had a party for my dad, and I ate a lot of junk and got a bit drunk. My bowels got blocked and pushed fluid onto my lungs, causing pneumonia. After they got me to A&E, my heart stopped. The doctors had to resuscitate me. They put me in intensive care and put me in an induced coma for three weeks, to treat the chest infection and monitor my recovery. After that, I had to spend eight to ten weeks on a respirator to build my respiratory health and restore proper bowel function.

I'm telling you this now because it gives a bit more context to what I'm about to say next. If you haven't experienced it, you won't quite understand just how much your life changes after an injury like this. Life was so hard, and so different, that for a long while after my accident, I was so focussed on just adapting to the changes, and being aware of the dangers, that I almost existed outside of myself. I had almost stopped thinking about myself as a physical being in a way. It didn't even occur to me that I hadn't seen myself in a mirror since before the accident.

Even after I had moved to a wheelchair, it was weeks before I realised that I had never looked at myself in it. In the early days of my recovery, I was simply too focussed on surviving, and then I began to realise that I had consciously avoided looking at myself. I wasn't ready to see myself in the chair, and I wasn't prepared to come to terms with the fact I couldn't get out of the chair and walk.

It was only when I was on a tilt table when I was in physio that I saw myself. There was a mirror in the corner of the room, and when I got back in my chair, I asked to take a look at myself. Somebody had been looking after my hair and my appearance all that time, but somehow it hadn't registered that I was not going to be able to take care of my own appearance again, and I was going to be reliant on somebody else to do it for me.

It's hard to really put into words just how it felt, but it was devastating. There was someone sitting in that chair I didn't quite recognise. The tracheostomy bag was like a part of me. That's when I finally knew just how helpless I was. It's one thing feeling helpless in your own body, but it's quite another thing to see it. To see and understand how helpless you have become. In that moment, you appreciate everything that the doctors have been telling you about how difficult life is going to be.

I didn't know then how I was going to get through day by day, never mind the rest of my life. You don't just see the chair, you see that you've been stripped of your freedom. It feels like a sharp shock of recognition, knowing that everything has changed, and you're embarking on life in a wheelchair.

I freely acknowledge that it took me a long time – certainly too long – before I could see myself as I really was. Everyone is different of course, but I would encourage anyone reading this who is in that situation to start looking in the mirror sooner. Like splitting up from my partner, or a loss in the family, you may well struggle to come to terms with it at first. But there comes a point where you have to accept what has happened. You learn to accept who you are, or you just can't carry on. You can't enjoy the rest of your life. There's no time limit on that. For me, it seemed as if everything happened at once, I lost my partner, the business was failing without me, and it took me eight or nine months before I felt ready to start making something more out of my life.

I should point out that, at the time of writing this, I am extremely comfortable with myself and my appearance. As with so many other aspects of my recovery, I didn't ever really think that would be the case.

I still had a long way to go with accepting myself for who I was, and I was going to be doing a lot of work with Katherine and Samantha, the nutritionist, over the months and years to come....

Andy (Mentor Support):

One of the most important things that I do for spinal cord injured people and families is giving them information about what is likely to happen next in the rehabilitation process, and what's likely to happen when they go home. It's really important at this stage for us to focus on the possibilities. There really are so many positive things that you can still do that will help you to move on in the right direction

Joe was in the spinal unit for quite a long time, and by the time he was getting close to leaving, we had developed a strong friendship and working relationship. I kept in touch when he went home to see how he was getting on, and I went to some of the events he put on that he'd talked about during his rehabilitation, including the all-day event at the Peace Hall in Halifax where he put on a fundraising event to raise money for Quad-Rebuild. This event was featured in the local newspaper and featured on ITV's Calendar programme. It was genuinely amazing. In all honesty, I thought he'd bitten a bit more off than he could chew, and I was astonished that he managed to pull it all off so well, but I shouldn't have been – Joe has absolutely amazing grit and determination.

Katherine (Neuropsychologist):

We do have to be mindful that even if hospital or a spinal unit can feel like a strange, unreal environment, getting out comes with its own pressures too. I have worked with people who have struggled to adjust to leaving the safe confines of the ward. Heading out into the real world and learning to live life in a completely different way, adjusting to being in a wheelchair, or being dependant on other people feels like a scary prospect. So it can be a very useful time to bring some psychology into play.

Sam (Joe's Sister)

When he came home, things started to change more quickly. It was hard for him in the hospital because we could only ever visit for so long, and he felt a bit isolated at times. Being left on your own is when the negative thoughts really start to build. But when you're home with your family, there's someone there all the time, just like there is for most of us. Or at work, there's someone we can talk to. Just having people around is a kind of medicine. Being able to go and visit people helped him to start to relax.

Barry (Joe's Friend):

His parents helped him set up round the clock care to look after him when he was discharged, but he spoke to them like he spoke to his lads on site. One by one they left, or they complained to the management. But after the accident, Joe couldn't control it. They soon parted company, and then they had to find a new care team. Joe being Joe didn't take any blame for that. Joe has calmed down a lot, but let's face it, for a very long time, he was an angry young man. He had every right to be an angry young man.

Peter (Joe's Dad):

We can't fail him. There have been times when he's wanted us to leave him alone, or he says, 'just let me die', but we're there for him, and we're ready to help when he needs us. Sometimes, that's all you can do as a parent, you sit and wait till they're ready.

11 Managing Food and Weight

After his injury, Joe's relationship with food changed. Bereft of the comfort of close personal contact, and unable to express his passion for stone carving, he sought solace in other ways.

After injury, you look for pleasure where you can find it. And I found it in food.

Joe:

> They say you have to rebuild yourself physically before you can begin to rebuild your image. Sure enough, my weight plummeted after the accident. I was about 70 kg before the accident, and I went down to about 55 kg. I obviously went without solid food in intensive care and when they brought me round – and for some time afterwards – I looked really gaunt in the face.

Samantha (Nutritionist):

> Many patients will be tube-fed while they're in intensive care or on a high dependency unit. People invariably lose weight when they have any kind of spinal injury as the body goes into shock following the traumatic injury, and that pushes the body into a catabolic state. So, nutrition will be an integral part of their journey towards improvement and/or recovery.
>
> After the initial acute phase following the injury, people generally go on to a rehab facility in a hospital or return home, depending on the severity of the injury and the support available. Usually by that point, the body will have adjusted to the injury, and their metabolic rate slows down, and their energy requirements reduce, and they suddenly find that they start to put weight on. It doesn't help that after an injury of that magnitude and the weight loss that goes with it, patients may often think: I need to put a bit of weight back on, only to find that it goes on a little too easily.

DOI: 10.4324/9781003430728-13

Joe:

When I got onto the rehab unit and was allowed proper food, I quickly got the taste for it again. I ate and ate in hospital – there was no end of sausage rolls in hospital and ice cream – and I carried on eating when I got out. I wanted more of the food that I liked, and everyone was happy to let me have it. I had almost died after all, so who was going to deny me when I asked for more and more snacks, or fry-ups. I wanted all of the food that wasn't good for me, and lots of it.

It was a lonely world after my injury. There wasn't anyone I could really share my experience with, and I was comfort eating. I was filling a hole and eating out of depression. I had lost the everyday, ordinary comfort of being able to cuddle my partner, or hug a friend. The satisfaction I had got from stone carving was lost to me. In the old days, I had been able to totally lose myself in the stone carving; I'd be in another world. What do you do when those things are taken away? You look for pleasure where you can find it. And I found it in food.

My weight went up to the point that I was filling my chair out. I looked at myself in the mirror one day when I was getting ready for an event, and something clicked inside me. I didn't like what I saw. It wasn't because of the chair this time, it was because I knew I had let myself go. My weight had gone up to 82 kg, and I knew that was a really substantial amount of weight gain. Obviously, it affected my mood; I'd always been a bit vain, and I'd always said I would never allow myself to get fat, but how do you lose weight when you're in a body that's not even able to move? If you have one small thing that isn't good for you, you know that fat is just going to come straight back.

Samantha (Nutritionist):

Joe's case manager, Katie, got in touch with me about Joe because he was keen to lose a bit of weight to help reduce his risk of cardiovascular disease. We know that patients with spinal cord injuries are at higher risk from cardiovascular disease, and of course being overweight is also a risk, and he was very aware of the health implications.

We all know that physical activity burns calories, so if you're less physically active, you need fewer calories, and inevitably, less food. That can be a hard lesson to learn and stick to. Lots of us eat food because we enjoy it, not necessarily because we're hungry. So that is the challenge for someone like Joe, who isn't able to be physically active, and his energy requirements are very low. Just a couple of 'naughty' meals can quickly undo the rest of his good work.

Joe:

I used to eat shit and then I felt bad about myself. It was a vicious cycle, because then I'd get depressed and eat even more shit. Seeing myself filling out my chair was a wake-up call. So even before I met Samantha, I worked hard on my own to try and lose that weight. I knew that would start to help me to feel good about myself again.

Samantha (Nutritionist):

I'm here to help people understand how maintaining optimal weight and good nutrition will help them mobilise more easily. I want people to understand exactly what their bodies need to give them the best chance of effective ongoing rehabilitation. We can see how managing weight and nutrition can significantly improve people's rehabilitation goals; they will feel better equipped to carry out weight-bearing activities, and will find physiotherapy easier to engage in.

In other words, we're not the food police, we're not here to tell anyone that they're fat or that they're making wrong choices, the dietary advice that we decide upon will be integral to somebody's whole rehab. Together we will find out what your body needs to be the best it can be.

I knew that Joe had been successful in losing a bit of weight by himself, but he was concerned about the overall nutritional balance of his diet, and wanting to feel like he was doing the best he could to maintain his overall health.

Joe:

The one thing more than anything that spurred me on was wanting to be a role model to people, and prove that just because you've got a spinal cord injury and so many impediments that restrict your daily living, it doesn't mean you can't still have an amazing life…

Samantha (Nutritionist):

That's the kind of information I want to hear. When I meet someone for an initial assessment, we take an hour and a half to get to know the person and the journey they've been on from a healthcare perspective, and a dietary perspective. Many people have tried to lose weight and struggled. Many people have been successful and then tipped back into old habits. So, it's important for me to understand the journey you've been on, what you've tried in the past what has been helpful and not so helpful, and what you're aiming to achieve. My job then was to do what I could to help Joe achieve that amazing life he spoke about.

Part of my initial assessment would include looking at activity levels, and I would use that to estimate a person's nutritional requirements. It all comes down to maths at the end of the day! To lose weight, we need to aim for 200–300 calories below their estimated daily requirement for maintaining their current weight. If they can stick to that, they/you will achieve weight loss. In Joe's case, I looked at meal plans based on those requirements, taking into account his requirements for protein, fibre, and a sufficient intake of vitamins and minerals.

I will also find out what your life is like now, and what your routine is like, how food fits into your life now, whether you go to work, or college, whether or not your drive, or exercise; all of these different things will have an impact on eating and accessibility to food.

It's also important for me to get to know any support staff that you might have, so I know what hours they keep, and if any of them have any particular interest or existing skills in food preparation; we can provide training for support staff to help them help you.

I will also need to look at what kitchen equipment you have, so I can tailor any suggestions that I make about preparing, cooking, and storing meals. The suggestions I make will also fit in with how easy or difficult it is for you to get shopping, and how often you or someone else goes shopping.

All of these little elements help me build up a picture of your normal routine so that whatever I suggest can fit in quite seamlessly to how you live, and what practical challenges you face on a daily basis.

We'll look at your wider life too; if you go out for drinks or meals with family and friends, or if you eat at other people's houses; all of these things will impact on food choices and nutrition and need to be factored into the work that we do.

My report will make recommendations for the ways in which I can help, and this will be as individual as the people I work with. Joe was very clear that he wanted some meal plans, so I developed some sample plans, and he reviewed them, telling me what he liked and what he didn't like. I revised it, and he tried it for a few weeks, and we went on tweaking it to make it as practical and as easy as possible.

Anyone with a significant spinal cord injury will obviously be completely reliant on their family and/or carers to support them in whatever dietary choices they make. You may be bound by what people can prepare for you, so it is really important that everyone involved is on the same page with regard to the work we're doing, and why we're doing it.

Sometimes we have to appear to be cruel to be kind. Understandably, family, friends, and loved ones are always very keen to take my patients out for a few meals, or bring them a few too many treats, when really it would be much better if they were to take them for a walk, or just pop over for a cup of tea. It's ingrained in our society – food is something you give when you love someone and you care about them, but sometimes, it can do more harm than good.

We will work with any support staff to support you in helping you achieve your goals, being mindful of repeating the training to accommodate staff turnover.

Gez (Carer):

Practically, it is true that carers will come and go. There isn't very much progression within the job, and nowhere else to go. Joe is fully aware that young people who come into the job with the ambition and drive are going to want to move on. At first it was hard for Joe to accept that, but as someone who has no shortage of motivation and drive himself, he understands that people may want to move on to work in a hospital or elsewhere.

Joe:

One of the great difficulties is training people to help me because people do come and go so much. There is a vocational aspect to some of these roles, and it's important that you try to find people to support you who really understand the demands (as well as the rewards) of the job.

Mary (Joe's Mum):

It's difficult when carers come and go. Emotionally it's hard: we meet them, we get to know them, and then they move on. We feel like they become a part of the family. And then we have to start all over with the new carers. And every time we have to go through so many of the same things that they need to know about Joe, and his food, and his safety. Of course, Joe always knows more about his condition than they do, and he can tell most of them a thing or two about nutrition.

Joe:

On a normal day, I'll have a bit of porridge for my breakfast, some soup, a baked potato or some fruit. For my dinner, I might have half a chicken breast with some potatoes and vegetables. It's advisable to eat small quantities every three hours or so. Sometimes, I might let myself have a mixed grill, or some junk food, but it's hard not to feel guilty afterwards. Even though I've lost all that weight, and even though I eat so carefully, I don't ever want to slip.

Samantha (Nutritionist):

I do ask that if you are helping, caring, or supporting someone, just listen to what they want. If they are keen to make dietary changes, you can really help them by respecting that choice and helping them to follow through on those choices, without imposing your own opinion on it, no matter how well-meaning.

As an add-on to that, I would say that if you are going to read around and Google things to try and help, do look at who has written that article or that paper so that you know it has come from a reputable source. There is a lot of badly researched or misinterpreted dietary information out there! It's very easy to do more harm than good. Ultimately, Joe was mostly driven by his own sense of who he wanted to be…

Joe:

Every day now, I look in the mirror. I make sure that I am happy with my appearance. I want to feel and look like my best self when I am meeting new people and going to events. That is where my motivation comes from

As I write, I'm down to 62 kg. I know that not everyone will care about their weight, but it was important for me to show that even if you are in a chair for the rest of your life with little or no movement, you can still take pride in your image and look after your weight. There are ways to do all of these things, and I wanted to prove that by example. I have also seen the better quality of life you can get from eating healthily and being proactive; how it can really give your mindset a boost. It's really important that you're getting the right nutrition in your diet, all the vitamins and minerals to maintain your bone density. You need regular carbohydrate foods to maintain your blood glucose levels. There's a fine balance between what you should and shouldn't be eating.

Samantha (Nutritionist):

Joe is absolutely right. In the NHS, a lot of people are referred to a dietitian by their consultant, and it isn't necessarily something that they see as a priority at that time. It can take a bit of explanation to clarify the role of a dietitian; that we look at overall nutritional care, it's not always specifically just about weight loss, it can focus on making sure the patient is getting the right mix of vitamins and minerals so your body can fight infection. Particularly for someone like Joe, with a high-level spinal cord injury, a chest infection can be really dangerous, so it's important to maintain good nutrition and overall health is an absolute priority.

I'm not here to judge my patients on their choices, it's much more important that we can work through these things together so that I can understand what drives their choices. And if it is the comfort that food gives that you're looking for, it might be time to reassess where that feeling of comfort really comes from. Often the comfort really comes from the people you're with. It's easy to associate the comfort we get from going out with a friend and having a coffee and a cake to the calories, when it is probably rather more about the company. If you had that same piece of cake at home on your own, it probably wouldn't taste as good. There are lot of examples of people eating because of the environment they're in, not because they're hungry. We do a lot of work with people helping them to tune into their bodies a little bit more to help them understand what their body needs.

For someone like Joe it is more difficult. The nature and severity of his spinal injury means that he doesn't get the same kind so sensations as most people, so he doesn't get the same sensations of hunger, or feelings of fullness. He is more of a visual eater, he will eat based on appearance and taste. But he really got into the specific target of aiming for a specific number of calories per day. He also wanted some flexibility with that, so we discussed how, if he wanted a treat one day, he could offset the calories against another day.

A lot of people realise that when they're on a diet, they will fall off the wagon at some point, particularly if they're following a really strict diet. That's just normal human behaviour. But they often find that when they have that treat – when they have that piece of chocolate cake or whatever it is – they very often realise it didn't actually taste that good anyway. Or people say the sense of guilt they felt around eating it meant that they didn't enjoy it anyway. So how can we learn from that kind of experience? Actually, we get more pleasure from feeling proud of ourselves, knowing that we stuck to the plan and we lost the weight, than we would have got from the physical sensation of eating the food.

Joe:

For me, it was loneliness that made me eat. I don't want other people to feel that same kind of loneliness. Even if you're reading this book thinking you're alone, you're not. You can still be in control of your own destiny, and accept help from the many, many people out there who want to help you. You don't need to use food to replace things that you've lost.

Samantha (Nutritionist):

I know it can seem difficult to try and make these kinds of life-style changes. But I've done a lot of work in the field of behaviour change, and I've done a lot of additional training around having these kinds of conversations with people, and there isn't an easy answer. A lot of the work we do as dietitians really falls under the description of counselling and talking therapy. It often comes down to a very pragmatic conversation around the pros and cons: what are the benefits of sticking to a diet versus the benefits of not sticking to a diet? And which benefits are more important to you in the long run? These are some of the benefits of working with a dietitian.

Joe:

Not everyone can have access to a dietician, to ensure they have the right balance of vitamins and minerals, fats, fibre and carbohydrates every day. But through my Quad-Rebuild charity, we will help people access that kind of support.

Andy (Mentor Support):

A big part of my work is with people who won't necessarily get that same vast level of support from a spinal injury centre, and are linked into that service for life. Those people have the reassurance of knowing that they can pick up the phone any time they need to and get help, support or advice. The specialist support and education they get going through the spinal injury centre really does set them up for life. So if a person doesn't go through that process, it can be challenging for them to move on from their anger into a more productive phase of rehabilitation. That's why charities like the Spinal Injuries Association and others who help spinal cord injured people are so vital.

Joe:

Working with a dietician can help you towards whatever you want to achieve. But you have to be honest with them…

Samantha (Nutritionist):

If you're going to be embarking on this process with a dietitian, the simplest thing you can do to help them help you get the most out of the process is to be honest with them. Don't be tempted to tell the dietitian what you think they want to know. I would also urge you to keep an open mind, you might be surprised by how much your dietitian knows, not just about food, but about the whole medical picture. Whichever dietitian you work with will have spent four years in training and they will have studied physiology and pharmacology; they understand anatomy and the properties and potential side-effects of your prescribed drugs. They will take a whole-picture view of your situation, of which food is just one part.

It's important to find a dietitian with the right kind of experience, and it also needs to be someone who you feel comfortable working with. We talk a lot about personal things, so you have to be able to be open and honest with your dietitian. For example, in Joe's case, with his complex medical history, I would need to know about his bowel function, as that can be significantly affected by dietary changes. Don't be afraid to talk about poo! What goes in must come out, and we will ask you about poo.

I would also need to know about medication, as certain medicines can have a significant effect on digestion. I'll ask about fluid intake and alcohol consumption; any lifestyle questions that may be relevant.

I will normally be in touch every couple of weeks in the early stages so that I can monitor progress and assess the results. In Joe's case, his injuries made it quite hard to assess his weight. We worked on getting him some specialist scales that would make it easier for him to weigh himself at home. I also use an app that allows people to record what they're eating on a day-to-day basis, and then I can analyse that from a nutritional point of view. This also allows us to compare it with the meal plan to see how closely they followed the plan, and if they didn't follow it, we can then try and find out why, whether that was because they had a day out, they didn't have the right food in the house, or they just didn't like that meal. Again, I must stress, there is no judgement here. It's all about helping me to understand what drives the choices patients make so that I can help them as much as possible.

After that intense period of activity in my first few months with a patient we gradually scale it back as they begin to take ownership of their food choices. You might need to see me once or twice and then you'll be on board and ready to go without any further help from me. Or you might want a bit more attention. Either way, your dietitian won't make things too prescriptive. Some people like meal plans – that was something that Joe wanted to try so that he knew there were no discrepancies in what he was eating – but a lot of people find them to be too limiting or boring. For the most part, they will work on improving education and encouraging people to make their own choices on a day-by-day basis.

Joe:

Understanding how food and nutrition factored into my overall recovery helped me to make better choices. I wanted to enjoy my food, but I also wanted to feel good about myself; with Samantha's help, I felt like I was able to take back control. Now, I can enjoy what I eat. I can still have a treat or two, so long as I eat responsibly the next day, I can look after my appearance and my health.

As Samantha mentioned, getting a better understanding the psychology behind my choices was a big part in unlocking my relationship with food. I felt as if I was making progress in so many ways, but I still had a long, long way to go.

Don't get complacent. There were times on my recovery journey where I got frustrated because things didn't move forwards as quickly as I wanted. Eventually you realise that recovery is not a straight road, you keep doubling back on yourself. Sometimes you have to go back and deal with things that you thought you'd already dealt with. And sometimes, you have to face some pretty tough questions. If I thought I'd fully dealt with the past, and everything that had happened to me, I was wrong...

12 Working with a Neuropsychologist

In any recovery, there is a point at which it's tempting to think there are no more hurdles to overcome. But for many people, as Joe discovered, that's the point at which they have to embark on some of the most challenging work of all.

Without that focus on the mind, it's really difficult to overcome the difficulties you are facing.

Michaela (Joe's Sister):

We are all proud of Joe for everything he has achieved against the odds. But it's obviously still upsetting to see Joe when he is struggling with his mood. Knowing what he was, and who he was before the accident makes it all the harder. He had such big plans for his business, and he clearly had a head for it. It was gong really well, so it was absolutely devastating when it was all taken away from him in the accident. It wasn't just the business though, I know he'd been thinking about one day getting married and having children.

He has plenty of good days, but I'm sure he would be the first to admit, there are bad days too. There probably always will be. And I know that he suffers more with bouts of anxiety now.

Sam (Joe's Sister):

Joe had had a few episodes of anxiety before. It was never anything to do with his work, it was more emotional anxiety, particularly around relationships. But after the accident, as you'd expect, his anxiety has sometimes threatened to overwhelm him.

Sometimes an anxiety attack will hit, or he will feel so worn down by everything that he doesn't want to go on. Joe will ring me whenever he needs to, even if it is at one o'clock in the morning. I just try to calm him as much as I can, and remind him of all the positive things he's achieved. We talk, and even more importantly, I listen. Sometimes that's the best thing anyone can do. There are

DOI: 10.4324/9781003430728-14

times when he just needs to get some of it off his chest, and it is important for him to know he can do that whenever he needs to.

Sometimes I'll try and get him to go to a good place in his mind. I know that meditation is a good way to help take him out of the pain of the moment and refocus his mind. There are some good resources online and I used to give Joe links to videos he could watch, just to calm his mind a little bit. You're never trying to take away the pain, or deny its importance, you're just trying to give the person a break from the endless narrative of pain and exhaustion.

Joe:

When you have such a catastrophic injury, it's tempting to think *what's the worst that can happen to me now?* Unfortunately, the truth is that you are probably going to face more hurdles, and each one brings a new set of problems for you to deal with. I have had to deal with a lot of traumatic experiences over the last four years of my life to the point now that I suffer with significant PTSD. I have flashbacks about some of those times in hospital, and stress dreams about being cut or having my nails torn out. It's hard to get over some of those things and move forwards.

Every time I went into hospital, the doctors and nurses told me, it's fine, don't worry, you're in safe hands. And you trust them. But every new operation, and every new procedure couldn't help unbalancing me a little bit more. After everything I went through, I felt so raw from the experience.

Katherine (Neuropsychologist):

Of course, it is not at all surprising that Joe experienced increased anxiety after the accident, and it can be very helpful to try to tackle some of those feelings of anxiety early on in your working relationship with a psychologist. In some cases, we will need to do a lot of work around processing the trauma that a person has experienced. One technique that I have used to help in this regard is called eye movement desensitisation and reprogramming (EMDR) – this can be a really useful intervention to help take some of the heat out of the trauma memories as well as tackling any blocks to processing, on more of an emotional level. With Joe, I used the Flash technique which can be considered a precursor to EMDR and is a gentle way of introducing processing work. Individuals are invited to bring up a distressing memory, just briefly and then shift attention to a positive engaging focus (holiday, favourite music). They are then instructed to blink when the target word 'Flash' is said followed by a brief glimpse of the traumatic memory and then the cycle is repeated.

Joe:

I tried different techniques with my psychologist to reduce the flash-backs and PTSD, but the severity of my PTSD creates good and bad days. Trying the EMDR technique brought memories back that I didn't want to remember. EMDR is quite a vibrant in-your-face process; you look into the corner of a room flicking your eyes backwards and for-wards, left and right, while you bring a bad thought or memory to the forefront of your mind, to be replaced by something more positive.

Katherine (Neuropsychologist):

The theory of EMDR is that by encouraging an individual to bring up the trauma memory, you are then over-taxing the working memory and supporting an individual to move through the memory whilst listening out for any places an individual may become stuck. This process allows the brain to put a time stamp on the trauma rather than remaining actively on alert for further threat. It's a really useful way of taking the heat out of some of the memories or the beliefs people have around the source of their particular trauma.

Historically there has been a belief around EMDR that if you can't remember the event then it's not worth doing. But actually, a person's beliefs around the event do endure. For many people the effects of a trauma play out in flashbacks or nightmares or how they relate to those around them, all of which can really affect quality of life. So EMDR is a great tool for challenging those beliefs, allowing people to function a little more easily.

Joe:

I have a lot of physical challenges in my recovery: I'm paralysed from the neck down, I have a suprapubic catheter, which has be-come blocked on a few occasions, my bowels have blocked a cou-ple of times, and I've had chest infections; all things which have been detrimental to my state of mind as well as my body. So as well as having the correct nebulisers, following the right diet, and doing whatever exercise I can, so meeting Katherine, and working with psychologists has helped me feel reborn. For me, it was key to mak-ing my rehabilitation work. I found out that rehab wasn't just about rebuilding my physical health, it was about my mind and my mental health too. Without that focus on the mind, it's really difficult to overcome the difficulties you are facing.

Katherine (Neuropsychologist):

Let's take a step back. If you are going to be working with a psy-chologist, you might want to know a bit more about their role and what you can expect.

Psychology is useful at various stages of a patient's journey following an accident like Joe had. A spinal cord injury obviously has a massive impact upon an individual, in every area of your life: mobility, dependence, roles in life, sexual relationships, identity, social life, mobility and driving, everything. At different stages of recovery, people need different things.

The process will begin with a full assessment, from which they will develop an evidence-based plan for treatment. But there isn't a one-size-fits-all approach, interventions can vary widely.

I do understand that the prospect of working with any kind of psychologist might feel scary or intimidating, at least at first. I know it was like that for Joe. He had always had some very ingrained rules for life about being self-sufficient and not relying on others, so it wasn't easy for him to accept the sort of help that he needed. When I met him in November 2019, it was about two years after his accident, and at that time, he was still quite stuck in not being able to move forwards in some ways, and was masking any tiny hint of vulnerability.

Joe:

It's true that the thought of speaking with a psychologist was quite alien to me. Of course, Katherine cottoned onto that very quickly; she saw how driven I'd been, and how I was so used to being independent. She guessed correctly that I would have buried my head in the sand rather than deal with my problems. But when I relaxed into the process, I probably sounded like I was going at a million miles an hour. I just couldn't get everything out that I wanted and needed to talk about.

Katherine (Neuropsychologist):

When Joe understood the value of what we were doing, he embraced the process. Crucially, he set about everything he did with hope, which is a small but essential part of the skills you need to progress.

Joe:

I'm a positive person. I am very focussed on achieving what I want to achieve. You might not feel that positive, or maybe you're just not at that stage yet. You might even be reading this thinking *that's bollocks, things will never improve*! I can tell you that I have spent so many years grieving and suffering in silence, crying myself to sleep some nights, and not knowing how I was going to get through the next day.

I started to learn the importance of looking my problems square in the face. I've had to endure all of the impacts that my spinal cord injury has placed on me. At the end of the day, you can either bury your head in the sand, or you can choose to get up, get going, and do everything you can to live your life to the fullest. I had been sceptical at first, but I was beginning to see that the benefits of working with a psychologist are huge.

Katherine (Neuropsychologist):

One of the hardest things for Joe to deal with was the loss of his relationship with Michelle, as he mentioned earlier. I know that they had been very close, and I think that she had helped to contain him and support him in the first few months after the accident. But when that relationship unravelled, it left Joe struggling to cope with the reality of his situation. I do think the breakup catalysed a lot of the feelings that Joe had been having around all the losses he had suffered as a result of the accident. For as long as they had stayed together, she had helped to mask some of that pain and kept him positive. So, when that deteriorated, he was left with a huge psychological shock. Like any kind of trauma, that kind of pain is not easy to resolve, particularly when it beds in and becomes entrenched – as it had done with Joe.

He found the process of therapy harder to engage with at first, particularly as he was mired in the pain of his break-up and everything else at that point. We spent several sessions on purusing the question of how he was going to move on without her. A lot of our work at first focussed on how he was ruminating on his relationship. At the time he was numbing himself with work, and of course, Joe has always been – and remains – fiercely driven in so many ways. His hard work and creativity, exemplified by his plans for his charity, the university studies he was embarking on, and his great drive to support people with this book were – and are – really laudable. But, on top of his building work, there was no time left for himself. And of course, that meant that he wouldn't think or feel as much about some of those difficult thoughts. He preferred to numb the feelings rather than sit with any of those distressing feelings.

We looked at developing his coping strategies and identifying his strengths since the accident, and we worked on enabling him to sit with those feelings of distress and work though them, rather than trying to numb them out of the way. Joe found himself caught between two extremes. On the one hand, he was absolutely determined to push forwards and do as much as he could to prove that he was still himself, but on the other he was burning himself out, getting exhausted, and found himself inconsolably sad and crying. He was caught between those extremes.

Developing coping strategies for those times when life feels overwhelmingly difficult is important for many of the people I work with. In particular, the work we did on distress tolerance was really key in helping Joe to deal with some significant issues.

We worked on helping Joe to identify some of the vicious cycles he was getting himself into. For example, he would often contact his ex and express his anger, and then the communication between them would stop, and he would feel remorse and apologise. Only for the cycle to begin again.

That led us into exploring the idea that we can't avoid difficult life events, whether they're break-ups or the kind of trauma that he had been through, but we need to be aware of the many things that we do that inadvertently prolong our suffering. It's easy to slip into ways of thinking that worsen how we feel, as expressed by Joe's punitive rumination. It's like washing old laundry, it keeps going round and round. Whatever the situation, whatever the source of stress, the question is: how do you tolerate something that you can't make better?

To answer that question, we can look at other areas of your life where you draw upon strength and perseverance, and you look at ways in which you can use those same skills and attributes to support you through it. And Joe did. In our discussions in sessions, he started to move away from his pain around losing his relationship to expressing general pain about the difficulties inherent in his new life, and the losses that he'd had to deal with.

Joe hadn't ever allowed himself the time for reflecting on his thoughts and feelings to that extent before. Even though he found it hard to give himself the time and space to think about these things, and missed a few sessions, he began to engage more and more with the work. (If you are finding the thought of exposing yourself to so many difficult feelings hard, then I can reassure you that it starts to feel easier and more natural as our time together goes on.)

Joe:

Katherine really helped me to be able to deal with my frustrations. Specifically, we worked on helping me to take a step back and look more objectively at what's going on in my life so that I can identify the good and bad parts more clearly. I had to learn to identify the reactions and responses that were available to me in response to something happening. I used to be really impulsive. If something bad happened, I got angry. I took all of my frustrations out on my friends and family or the nurses. I was turning into somebody that nobody liked.

Katherine helped me understand how my mind works so that I could put coping mechanisms in place that would distract me away from harmful and hurtful thoughts and feelings. That was important, because you get to a point where you just can't live with those kinds of destructive thoughts all the time. I needed a break from them, and I needed to learn how to take responsibility for that. So I learned how to defuse difficult situations, take deep breath, refocus and carry on with my day.

Katherine (Neuropsychologist):

As time has gone on, Joe has become more and more interested in understanding the role of compassion towards himself, and others, in aiding his recovery. Understandably, Joe has experienced a lot of anger and managing that. Before the accident, he did have good coping strategies; he derived a lot of satisfaction from his creativity, his work, and his relationship with his girlfriend, and he met a lot of his psychological needs that way. But post-accident, there were times when his anger threatened to overtake him. We identified that not showing himself the necessary compassion was a real barrier to letting him tune into his distress and then be motivated to do something to reduce it.

Joe:

Working with a psychologist in the hospital helped me to start shifting my mindset, but it wasn't until I started working on my distress tolerance – my ability to withstand difficult situations – with Katherine that I learned how to channel my frustrations and energy without upsetting myself or getting angry. I take my hat off to anyone who is learning to deal with something like this – whether it's a spinal cord injury or something else – there are frustrations that are out of your control at every turn. A big part of distress tolerance is re-training the way your mind responds so you learn to accept the things that are not in your control. It means taking a step back. Practically that might mean waiting a day before replying to a message that has upset you. And it means being kind to yourself.

Every time I need to go into hospital again, it feels like another test of my coping strategies. The flashbacks return and my distress levels rise, so I have to try and channel that energy and redirect my brain. Everyone will find their own way, but for me, the easiest way to deal with it is to shift my attention onto my work or my charity; they are my driving passions. That is what helps to keep me focussed. This isn't necessarily easy to do, but a psychologist can really help you to shift your attention in a way that works for you.

Barry (Joe's Friend):

> I know there have been dark thoughts, I know there have been times when he has cried himself to sleep, but he has amazing resilience. He seems to be able to take the most extraordinary setbacks in his stride.

Katherine (Neuropsychologist):

> Joe has shown incredible resilience, but inevitably, there have been times in his journey when life has felt almost overwhelmingly difficult. If you are reading this, and you are concerned about your own state of mind – or you are worried about your friend or loved one – I do promise you that there is hope, as Joe has amply shown.
>
> From a professional point of view, it is important to know that a thorough risk assessment is an integral part of the process for every client. And it might sound counterintuitive, but actually talking to a patient about any thoughts that they have had around suicide and getting it all out in the open can be helpful; it actually reduces the sense of shame that people have.
>
> We will look at people's levels of hopelessness versus hopefulness, and what reasons people have for living. We'll consider people's ability to problem-solve. Of course, we are always looking for any potential red flags, but also intervening and collaboratively managing suicide through interviews, through contracts, safety plans and more to help contain someone at their lowest ebb. We would go on monitoring risk regularly, and have a very clear escalation plan so that everyone knows what to do and what services to involve if there are any concerns around people's safety.
>
> We also need to be aware that there are a lot of secondary drivers to suicidality that can be addressed. I can't overstate just how debilitating persistent pain and sleeplessness can be following an injury of the severity that Joe had. Good interventions to target these secondary drivers can really help in terms of improving people's sense of hope.

Joe:

> It's incredible what you can learn to deal with. It really is. It's a hard lesson to learn, but who you were before is gone in a way. You have to accept that, and adjust your mindset so that you can get the most out of your relationships and your life. It all comes back to distress tolerance and learning how to make these adjustments so that you can make the shift from hospital to home, and the shift from reacting to things in a negative way to a more positive way. It's about balancing the forces that act against us so that we can live as fully and as independently as we can.

Once you have accepted what has happened to you, the work begins on channelling and redirecting your energy in new ways. From working with Katherine, I know that you can step back and, channel all that energy in a different way. It's taken me a long time to get to that point, to be able to look at some of these situations from a different angle.

Think about how you can actually benefit from what has happened. For me, the major benefit has been the opportunity to give something back; to help people who may be struggling with the new life they are facing up to. I've heard of people who have survived cancer, or survived a near-death injury or experience who want to give back to their community; they feel compelled to do it.

I want to help people turn that negative into a positive. To guide and mentor people, to help them adapt and build their rehabilitation from the ground up. Through classes and workshops, we'll look at what impedes individual progress after injury and look at how people can transcend their impediments.

Even if you have had a high-level injury, you can still adapt and carve out a new life for yourself. You don't have to find a new vocation. There may still be job opportunities out there that will work for you, or even volunteering opportunities. The important thing is that you find your way of living the life you want to the fullest.

Katherine (Neuropsychologist):

Joe is absolutely right that life can improve in many, and in surprising ways. Of course, a lot of the work you do with your psychologist will take place over time, and it may represent ongoing work that you will always be engaged on. It does takes time for new ideas to bed in, and for you to embrace new ways of thinking and behaving. For example, I have spoken to Joe about noticing when he is pushing forwards with too much urgency, as if he is aiming for a finish line that just isn't there. Pushing yourself too hard like that will just lead to burnout. What we try to encourage instead is pushing forwards with a greater emphasis on mindfully noticing the steps you are taking.

Of course, I understand how, at the start of the process, it can be really tempting to try and do everything all at once. Joe wanted me to explain to him the strategies he needed so he could push ahead and reach his goals quicker. I needed to encourage Joe to be a bit more curious about how he was feeling about what was in his mind, rather than him trying to *fix it*. It is important to try and foster a sense of curiosity about your thoughts, rather than letting them slip into judgement and criticism. Then we can think more about how to support you in alleviating some of your distress.

It was a challenge for Joe to be a bit more still, but he has begun to put some clearer boundaries in place so that he doesn't work after a certain time at night, and he does take time off at the weekend.

Michaela (Joe's Sister):

If there is one major thing that Joe is incapable of, it's sitting down and relaxing! And that has really helped him to keep going after his accident. He's always been a person on the go, and he'd find it impossible to do nothing. Before the accident, we had to tell him to slow down sometimes. Today Joe is determined to show people that in spite of everything that's happened, and in spite of his injury, you can still be successful, you can still (pretty much) lead a normal life, or as near to normal as possible.

Katherine (Neuropsychologist):

Slowing down remains a work-in-progress for Joe, and it might be like that for you too. Joe started to put the brakes on slowly at first, and then began to increase the balance between work and leisure activities. In his case, he decided to learn Spanish, and he started to watch some series on Netflix. Even something as simple sounding as setting aside a couple of hours to watch TV really helped him to make a qualitative difference.

Employing a PA, has had a really positive impact on him too. He knows that he can trust her to take so much responsibility off his shoulders. She has helped to contain him too, encouraging him to pull back from working too hard. While it might not be appropriate for you to have a PA, it can be a huge help to have someone in your life that is able to reduce some of the practical burdens that might cause you unnecessary stress.

Hayley (PA):

Joe had a few PAs before me, and I think it might not have been the best time for him, what with everything he was having to deal with at that time, not least of which was recovering from his accident. But as time went on, and he knew he wanted to do more and more, including establishing the charity, and then starting on a university degree, he found that he needed help with so many different aspects of his life.

It was clear that he wanted someone who could do more for him than handle his correspondence and administer his affairs, he wanted someone to help him drive what he wants to achieve, and someone who would share in his values and enthusiasm to get things done. My background was in charity and events work so I have been able to give him that peer-level support.

Katie (Senior Case Manager):

One of the most important learning points for Joe has been learning to take on board other people's advice. Remember where he was and what he was achieving on his own before the accident – it can be hard to surrender that complete autonomy and re-learn how to listen to other people's ideas and advice, based on their experience. Joe recognises that other people's knowledge – where they have particular experience that he doesn't – is really worth listening to so that he can make the most informed decisions. And I have really seen that develop in Joe.

Joe:

There's a balance between finding independence and leaning on others, like my PA and carers for support. It took me a while to reach that point, but working with Katherine really helped. I didn't appreciate how significant it was going to be for me to work with a psychologist, and how reassuring it's been to have someone there to talk to. But as I've gone on working with Katherine, I've gone on to appreciate how much she has encouraged me to be as self-sufficient as I can be. If you start off learning all you can from the people who are there to help you, you will go on to find the things that work for you and help you to feel more independent again.

I got to the point where I was able to accept the new me; it was like starting from step one. And that's the journey that I want to talk about with people. That's the message that I want to spread: don't take anything for granted. Don't waste the time you've got; try and make the most of each minute you've got.

Life can get better. It can even get better than it was before in some, if not in many ways. I feel as if I have a greater appreciation of life. The drive to help other people has helped me to look at life through a different lens.

13 Up, Up and Away

Joe and his family were always told be realistic in terms of what they could expect of his recovery. But that didn't stop him pushing as hard as he could for even more improvements.

The technology is amazing... The things they can do now have opened up all sorts of new possibilities.

Rachael (Neuro Physiotherapist):

They say, 'it takes a village,' and I think, as the contributors to this book have made clear, one of the secrets to effective rehabilitation and therapy is building a knowledgeable team who can offer support in many and varied ways, and help you lead a fulfilling life. The more people you have working for you who can open out possibilities for you, the better, both in terms of maximising physical potential, but also in terms of working with you to reach for – and attain – your goals.

The risks of respiratory deterioration, of joint range and postural issues, and many other issues across the spectrum of physical and mental health are too much to address on your own. Being well-managed means you are far less likely to get ill and pick up avoidable complications.

Katie (Senior Case Manager):

Joe had a definite need for physiotherapy, and assistance in accessing technology. At the time, he was completely reliant on his carers and PAs to help him with every type of communication, whether it was business-related or private, and it was obviously very difficult for him not to have any privacy whatsoever. It was really important to give him some sense of independence with that.

Rachael (Neuro Physiotherapist):

In our work, I provide a range of traditional physiotherapy, which looks at maximising a range of movement, maintaining postural

DOI: 10.4324/9781003430728-15

alignment, chest physiotherapy and respiratory management, maintaining or optimising respiratory function. But we also have an emphasis on accessing technology, including muscle stimulators, tilt tables, bikes, and all the technological adjuncts to therapy, as well as specialist clinic services.

One of the most important features of our work is in helping people maximise access to their environment, a good example of this would be helping people to stand using a standing wheelchair. We will also maintain opportunities for access to future development in rehabilitation to accommodate people's needs as their rehabilitation – and their competencies – develop.

It's a person-led approach, so we're very focussed on helping people to achieve their own goals. Knowing what they're hoping to be able to do helps to direct our focus. Of course, we're directed by a clinical assessment too. During an assessment you'll be asked to tell us about the issues and challenges that are facing you, and we will look at what function you have available, what range of motion you have, and consider any future risks. We want to minimise the risk of developing contractures or preventing chest infections, and we'll certainly consider cardiovascular risk. Working with Joe, for example, it was important to look at ways in which he could maintain cardiovascular health, even though he doesn't have active control over his muscles. It is important that you can still achieve some of that metabolic effect without being able to do those kinds of movements voluntarily.

As everyone has said, and I concur, Joe is certainly quite a driven individual, and from the start, many of his goals were around being able to access the community and take part in life as fully as possible. So, his priorities included being able to access any new technology that came along as his recovery progressed, and being able to progress to standing. We worked on maintaining his range so that he was able to use a standing wheelchair, making sure he could manage his blood pressure when moving into standing.

Underlying everything, we had to try to ensure that he stayed in the best possible physical shape to enable him to do the many, many things he wants to be able to do. As part of this work, we paid special attention to his respiratory function, and his care staff were carefully trained to do all of the things he needed to do on a daily basis when I'm not there to help him to remain healthy. That includes chest management and joint and muscle health, as well as range of movement exercises, passive exercises and setting Joe up on the equipment we've provided such as his tilt table.

Joe has a 'Functional Electrical Stimulation' bike which stimulates the muscle at the motor point and contracts the muscles so that

Joe can do active cycling despite his spinal cord injury. Of course, physiotherapy shouldn't just be something that you do occasionally, it needs to be built into your normal day-to-day routine. So, the care staff work with Joe on the tilt table every day, which progresses from a horizontal to a standing position so that we can move towards a standing wheelchair.

Peter (Joe's Dad):

The technology is amazing. You never know what's going to happen over the next few years. The things they can do now have opened up all sorts of new possibilities for Joe, and for others.

Ross (Joe's Friend):

Right at the start, the doctors told us we had to be realistic in terms of what improvements Joe could make. In a way, they were right to be cautious; we're more limited now in terms of what we can do and where we can go, but we've still been able to go out for a few meals, and I know that Joe wants to come out and have a drink with us, like he used to. So I think he has already achieved more than any of us thought would be possible.

Mary (Joe's Mum):

We're just try to stay hopeful there will be even more improvements. So much has changed since Joe's accident. There were so many things they said Joe would never be able to do again. There is talk of getting him off his vent for a few hours at a time in the future. He already uses the running machine, which moves his limbs for him, and it's amazing to watch him use that. There are things out there that can help to stimulate the muscles, and there is even hope that he might be able to get in a special kind of bath that would help him to feel his limbs. We're hoping he will be able to use a standing wheelchair. All his mates go out drinking, but most of the time, he can't go. So that would help him to feel more independent.

Rachael (Neuro Physiotherapist):

It's important that we are always really clear and realistic about what goals we're setting. Depending on what people's aspirations are, we can look at how we move towards that goal, even if may not always be in the way that a person would imagine. For example, if someone wants to cycle in a big run, they may not compete in the way they imagined, but we will try to find ways to help them access those kinds of experiences. One of our clients wasn't able to walk, but wanted to do the Great North Run! We pushed him around the route, and then stood him up to take him over the line. While they didn't have the complete experience of competition, they did engage in many of the elements that anyone competing in the run would experience. They still experienced a lot of the same challenges and rewards of taking part. So it is important that we are able to work towards finding alternative ways to help people move towards their goals.

Joe's level of injury is obviously quite significant, so in terms of functional change, we were looking at how we could support the access to the things he wants to do. Joe really is a testament to one of the great truths of this process: as described above, there is very often a way to do things that nobody has really thought about before. So it's important that we are always creative in thinking around the steps of that process working back from the ultimate goal to see what we are working towards and what steps we need to do to support that. So, if we are working towards somebody going out for a drink with their friends, we might think about accessing a standing wheelchair, using splints, or working on specific movements with their support team, all depending on the level of their injury. There can be a whole host of things that give the person a sense of moving towards their outcome goals.

Even when the work is hard and the road to achieving goals may seem like it's a long and winding one, there are moments when you can stop and realise just how far you've come. We can use one of Joe's goals as an example. It is, on the surface, quite a simple goal of being able to stand at the bar with his mates and have a drink. As with all goals, it helps to break it down into discrete parts. It's the muscles that keep your blood pressure up when you stand up, so that presents a challenge when you don't have active muscle control. We have done work with Joe on the tilt table on maintaining standing, moving from a very low tilt towards full tilt. And when he can maintain the standing stance at full tilt, then we know we will be able to try a standing wheelchair. Joe is very close to being able to do that and it is a great marker of progress.

As Mary mentioned, the technological developments over the last ten years have been tremendously progressive, and have the potential to take the physio process to a whole new level. There is an exoskeleton which is like a robotic suit that the person gets into. There are treadmills that they can be strapped into. These kinds of tools help create a pattern of walking, which really aid the rehabilitative process. They allow some people to make multiple movements in the kinds of patterns that can eventually mean they can move the limbs themselves, independently. For those who may never be able to move independently, these things still allow them to access those movement patterns which still provide excellent work for the body.

If you're going to be working with a physiotherapist, rest assured that everything they do will be built your very specific needs. Your physio will create a programme for you to engage in every day. For example, if you need support in moving your limbs to ensure they don't lose range in the joints, you will need to work on a daily programme. It isn't just about exercise, it's about considering how you sit and how your body is positioned at rest so that joints don't get tight in one set position. So we will build these things into the daily routine, whether that is with a device that exercises your arms and legs, or whether it's work that you're able to do yourself or with your carers or family.

It's important that we're all on the same page and working towards the same ends, so we work with carers and family to make sure they understand how to support you in the right way. And we work with you so that we can fit these things into your day in a way that works for you. In Joe's case, his carers can assist him in getting on and off the tilt table and the bike. They will assist him with his passive range of motion activities and respiratory physiotherapy to ensure that he is able to clear any chest secretions and ward off infections. Anybody with a higher-level spinal cord injury or any respiratory condition needs to take very special care of their chest management.

Barry (Joe's Friend):

Joe needed lots of practical adaptations to enable him to live in a way that gave him some more freedom. One of the first things I did was to build a removable ramp at my home so that he wouldn't have any reason not to visit. I put in an internal ramp on the other side so now Joe can go straight up to the door, and turn straight into the lounge. I think there was some reluctance from Joe's carers at first, so he left it a while before striking out on his own and visiting people, but Joe needed that escape. People do. I think it's really important to be able to go on visiting friends and family, and go living a social life so much as possible.

Rachael (Neuro Physiotherapist):

I will keep in contact with Joe indefinitely, so that I can problem solve any current issues and continue looking ahead to see if there are any new technologies or new processes that will help Joe. On my visits I will check posture, seating, and exercise performance. Ongoing access to therapy is really important to anyone with a neurological condition. It's important to manage the normal process of aging, which can necessitate revisions and adaptations to the techniques we employ. More than that, we are here to support people's ongoing goals, whatever they might be. Having said that, Joe did recently ask me about getting in a roller-coaster, and I might just have to delegate that elsewhere!

Barry (Joe's Friend):

My admiration for what Joe has achieved is boundless. He will not simply accept this is how it's going to be. He wasn't supposed to be able to do any of the things he can do now. A roller-coaster? A hot air balloon ride in your wheelchair? No problem for Joe.

Joe:

I wanted to show that I could live without too many compromises, and I thought that a balloon ride was a good way of showing just how much we can do, even with significant bodily restrictions. I was lifted into a bucket seat in the basket of the balloon, and was able to enjoy the freedom and the views, just the same as everyone else. As my recovery was progressing, it seemed a good way of illustrating that my trajectory was going up and up.

Rachael (Neuro Physiotherapist):

As you will have gathered, Joe is always pushing to see what he can achieve next, and he doesn't let things get in the way of pursuing his dreams. So when he said he wanted a supercar experience, nobody thought it would be possible, at first. A Lamborghini isn't a hugely practical vehicle for somebody with a complete spinal cord injury, and of course Joe can't drive himself anymore. Nevertheless, Joe and his care team arranged for him to be hoisted into a Lamborghini, and having hired it for a day, his friends drove him around in it.

So much of the work we all do is about finding creative ways around problems, and I have no doubt that Joe will go on presenting his team with new challenges to address and new goals to aim for. I think that is a really positive outlook for anyone. Essentially, therapy is really about achieving one's full potential, and that is certainly what Joe is doing and will go on doing.

Of course, everyone is different, and the psychological impact of a traumatic injury or an acquired injury affects people in different ways. If people are well-supported by the whole range of therapy, from psychological therapy, through to physiotherapy and all points in between it does smooth the transition into a different way of life. The challenge for people is when they are left to go home without any follow-up rehabilitative support, and if you feel as if you have not been getting the kind of support you need, then I would urge you to contact one of the bodies listed in this book who may be able to help you access more support.

And if you ever feel yourself flagging, if the work feels too onerous, or pointless, try to remember that none of the work you do will
ever be set just for the sake of it. Some of it is designed to maintain
your health and strength, of course, but the greater part of it will
usually be dedicated to helping you move towards your gaols. That
is why we invest so much importance in setting and sticking to clear
patient-centred goals.

I know that the work you have to do may be hard – and it may
be ongoing for a long period of time – but I think that when you're
clear about the goals you want to achieve, it will help you to focus
on doing that work and sticking to it. There will be markers along
the way that help us all to see that the work is being effective, and
that will help you to see and believe that you are moving towards
your desired outcome.

Above all, I do urge you to think about what extra support you
might be able to get to help you. That short stint in rehab in hospital
really is just the start, and if you look outside of what is available
in the NHS setting, there are more opportunities for you to access
specialists and technologies that will help you to make further progress. Joe's charity is a good place to start making your enquiries!

Andy (Mentor Support):

It's great to see how he's progressed. Inevitably, there were times
when we didn't get to meet up or speak quite so often; we were both
very busy. And when I did hear about him again, I found out that
he'd just come back from Barcelona! Wow! Again, I shouldn't have
been surprised. But those are the sorts of things we'd talked about
in rehab. Those are the sorts of things that people can go on and do,
even after an injury of the magnitude Joe had. It was wonderful to
hear that he'd done it, and I enjoyed hearing from him, how it had
all gone.

Joe:

Travelling abroad obviously isn't as easy for me as it used to be, but
I've still managed to go on many trips as a quadriplegic. Barcelona
was just the start for me, over the last few years, I've been to Corfu,
Cyprus, Lanzarote, Tenerife, and other places, and I'm always looking to find new places to visit.

It takes a bit more planning, but it can be done. By the time
I made it to Barcelona, I felt more than ready, and I had a good team
in place to help me – a mix of competent and non-competent staff.
(Competent staff are trained to deal with nebulisers, catheters and
can change a tracheostomy.) When I go away, I have to ensure that
I've got competent members of staff available day and night.

When I go away next, I'll be going for 12 nights with a team of four carers. Normally, you'd expect to need a team of six or seven carers, so everyone can have time off, but my carers are happy to manage the workload between them; we've found a way of doing it that works for all of us.

The airline will need to know what kind of wheelchair (and/or breathing apparatus) you're using, particularly as you can't put lithium batteries in the hold. There may be space restrictions governing the size of chair they can accommodate too. (You might need to get used to collapsing your chair so it meets the storage restrictions.) When I've travelled with Jet 2, I've had a very good service. (Other airlines are available, but they, in particular, have served me well.) See if your airline has special assistants to help you at check-in and with getting on and off the plane.

You'll probably be allocated a seat at the back of the plane, so that nobody can sit behind you and adjust your harness. You may need to be hoisted to your seat using a 'Crelling' harness which secures you safely into the seat with bucket straps under your bottom and over your shoulders. We strap my knees and arms together so they don't move around awkwardly. You may also want to use the pressure cushion from your wheelchair on the plane seat, as I do. If I'm flying for a few hours, we need to maintain my skin integrity. Every hour we get a bit of movement and get a bit of blood flow to the bottom. My carers will help with this, and I'll sit in the middle of an aisle of three with a carer on either side of me.

There are disabled access travel companies out there, but you may want to save yourself some money, and do a lot of the research yourself. The more research you can do upfront the better. A lot of places are not disabled-friendly. You need to check out the accommodation facilities, and the lie of the land around the hotel. Have a look on Google Earth and see if there any steep kerbs or hills that might make getting about in a wheelchair difficult? You may even need ramps to get up and down.

To help, I've set up a disabled access company, called Access the World, which will be working in conjunction with villas, hotels, lodges, flight operators, van hire companies and providers of hoists, commodes, and ramps. The aim is to create a one stop shop for accessing the world with a disability. You'll be able to get more information through the Quad-Rebuild website, steering you towards disabled friendly locations and doing a lot of the work for you. I've been to places that have claimed to be disability-friendly, but have been anything but. I want to try and improve your access to the world.

14 The World of Assistive Technology

The world of IT-related assistive technology is evolving rapidly, but finding out what sort of tools will help you – and learning how to use them – is half the battle.

Ultimately, it isn't about the technology, it's about belief. It's about finding ways for you, or your loved one to begin to interact in some way using technology.

Hayley (PA):

Technology really has been key in helping Joe; there are things out there that can help people to live more independently. For example, Joe can't physically write down the ideas as they come into his head, but he has learned to make the best use of apps and software, whether that's talking to Alexa (Amazon's voice-activated AI smart device that can answer queries and carry out a range of automated functions) or using Apple notes to record his ideas and get things done, voice control has been a real benefit. It's helpful knowing that if he needs anything in the middle of the night, he can use Siri to call someone straight away or ask Alexa in the bedroom to call the Alexa in the carers' staff room.

We communicate a lot using Groups, so he can interact with people, and talk to multiple people easily, and everything is available for him to review without him having to make notes. Zoom has been really useful for us too, and we can arrange group meetings so much more easily now. Joe wants to use his charity to make people aware of all of the things that are out there that can help – and make them accessible.

Sean (IT/Assistive Technology Consultant):

Joe can use eyegaze technology to achieve a lot of what he needs to do. Like a joystick, eyegaze is essentially an alternative mouse, but one that is controlled using the eyes. It's like magic technology, it's

DOI: 10.4324/9781003430728-16

the sort of thing that makes people go 'wow!' when they experience moving a mouse pointer around the screen with their eye movements. Eyegaze is really just a way of accessing the computer, but when it works for a person, it makes an excellent alternative to a mouse.

Sometimes it is the simplest things that yield the best results. I set up a computer for Joe to use with a screen mounted over his bed, and I gave his support worker a keyboard with an integrated touch-pad mouse, like one that you find on a laptop. She told me it was the best thing ever! Now, if Joe ever needs something doing, his support worker can access his screen through the keyboard and touch-pad mouse without having to lean over him. They don't even need to move his screen out of position to use the computer's touch screen, an act that can leave fingerprints behind, and be a potential distraction when using eyegaze. It was very simple, and it was very cheap, but it probably wouldn't have been top of anyone's shopping list when putting an eyegaze device in place!

Ultimately, it isn't about the technology, it's about belief. It's about finding ways for you, or your loved one to begin to interact in some way using technology. Technology might not be a button, it might be a piece of paper with letters on it. Don't consider anything to be insignificant, and remember that little developments can often lead to bigger developments.

*

I first met Joe following a referral from his case manager, Katie, and I accompanied her to see him, armed with some equipment. He didn't know about the potential for IT-related assistive technology to help him at that stage. He was particularly interested in the facility to position a screen so that he could see it more easily directly in front of him. I devised some ideas for how the assistive technology could help him. Seeing how he used his mobile phone when a support assistant presented it to him and then tapped the screen for him, I recommended and demonstrated how a Windows tablet set up using buttons controlled by his head, or eyegaze, would allow him to interact with the Windows screen himself so that he could access email and internet.

I left some of my kit with him, including a rolling floor mount, with an eyegaze-operated screen attached, which allowed adjustment to the position of the screen, so that he could try it out. A few weeks later, we discussed how he'd got on. He liked the functionality of the eyegaze system, but wasn't keen on the rolling floor mount – it's a wide based, large piece of kit that looks a bit like a small crane, and it didn't really fit in at his father's house where he was staying at the time. We talked about alternatives to that, and so I set up a device to attach the eyegaze to his wheelchair.

Following Joe's initial try-out of my equipment I recommended a Windows tablet, mounted and positioned in a way that he could access it easily using eyegaze. I configured it so that he could control it to access the computer features that he wanted. He also wanted to be able to control his Mac laptop, which at the time of writing is not possible using eyegaze. Instead, I set up computer-to-computer remote control software, which is freely available to individuals to use. It meant that Joe could see and interact with the Mac that his PA uses via his Windows tablet, using eyegaze.

I've continued to see him since then, just making sure that everything is alright and making any little adjustments. Now that he has moved into his new property, we expect that his needs will change.

Empowering as the technology is, we have to accept that fatigue plays its part, and like many people, Joe will still rely on care staff to do a lot of things. It's just more convenient to ask someone to pick up your phone and write a message to your friend sometimes, and Joe does like to get a lot of things done quite quickly! But I think that he has seen that, even if he doesn't want to do it all for himself all the time, he can do it. There are means and methods for him to do many of the things he wants to do.

I've put in place a couple of things to help him do as much for himself as he possibly can. I set up WhatsApp on his eyegaze machine, and I set up his online banking. He was very happy to be able to independently access his online banking, enter his own details, and access his accounts without ever having to ask a third party to do it. It was a practical advantage, but even more importantly, it's vital for people to be able to take back control of their own affairs and protect their online identity as much as possible.

*

So, how does the process of helping you find the right assistive technology work? When you, your case manager or representative gets in touch, I'll want to try and find out a little bit more about you, so that I can understand what challenges you're facing in the short and longer term. Timing is very important. You may have been in hospital or in a specialist unit, and your days will probably have been filled with various activities. But when you come home, there is often a bit of a lull, and that's when some despondency can set in that nothing is happening. So it makes sense to investigate whatever technology might be available to you as quickly as possible. I endeavour to be with someone within a week of their coming home.

I'll come and see you with my car full of equipment so that you can try different options that might be able to help you.

Following my first visit, I will write a report for you or your case manager making my recommendations for introducing any equipment, with additional recommendations for any training required to use it, not just for you, but for any family or carers that may also need to help.

If you have a solicitor working on your behalf, I (or your technology provider) can invoice them for the required kit. But it may be easier, quicker, and more cost effective for me to provide the kit and invoice afterwards. That way your solicitor won't have to charge you for making the correct purchases from the various equipment and software suppliers.

It may be necessary to introduce equipment over the course of several weeks or months, and it's important to review progress regularly to see how you get on with it. I do think you need to try the kit out, so I almost always recommend that you have a trial period to put it through its paces. It may be that it is the right equipment in the wrong setting, or it may be that a small variation or a tweak can enhance the experience and make it more useful to you. I'll set up weekly or fortnightly visits in the first instance so that I can work with the individual and work with the kit so they can really get to grips with it.

Having worked with a lot of people who live with a wide range of challenges, I can often draw on experience of what has worked for a person in a similar situation. It won't always be the expensive equipment that is most helpful. A speech and language therapist introduced me to a man who had been in a road traffic accident. Apart from a little movement in his arms, he had been left paralysed from the neck down, and he was unable to speak. He had already met with a technologist who had sold him thousands of pounds worth of kit, but its implementation hadn't been going very well. He hadn't benefitted from any of it in the ways that he had hoped.

As with Joe, he was only able to sit looking forward, and was unable to move his body to look around him, so he needed to have something in position that would work for the physical limitations he had. Sometimes it really is the smallest adaptations that can make the biggest difference; positioning and mounting the equipment is probably the most important thing in terms of making the equipment usable. So it's important to take the time to get these things right, or all the equipment in the world isn't going to help.

When you get started with eyegaze kit, for example, I'll set you up in front of the screen, and we'll adjust the positioning until it works for you. Eyegaze takes some getting used to – and it's not for everybody – but it can be really helpful for anybody who used a computer before the change in their life, as it has been for Joe. As with all of these things, the crucial thing is that you don't know if it might work for you until you try it. So it's important that you work with a technologist who will give you the time and the opportunity to try these things out.

To my other client, the eyegaze control of a computer was a game changer. Within about 25 minutes he was successfully using it to operate an on-screen keyboard to type messages and during that first session I also programmed the 'channel up' and 'channel down' controls so he was even able to experience using it to operate his TV.

Little victories like this can dramatically enhance someone's day-to-day experience, and make it so much easier to do some very important activities. Sometimes it takes just a single button to make a massive difference. Just think about what a huge difference it can make to somebody if they are able to press a button with their head or foot to operate a fan to cool themselves down on a hot day. I think it helps to demonstrate what is possible, and it says: this is just the beginning.

Wherever possible, I try to meet people's interests, perhaps they're interested in watching films, playing games, or listening to music, and I can factor that into what we do.

Interest in game playing is a good example as it's one of the most challenging things that many people may have enjoyed before an accident which seems almost impossible afterwards. It may be that I can help individuals to find ways to play computer games completely independently, or through collaboration with someone else. I can set up systems so that a person can perform one function using an item of assistive technology while somebody else performs another using a conventional game controller, thus including the person in a real gameplaying experience.

A lot of the kit I use can be employed to augment the communication of people who can't speak. However, I have found that communication can be low on any list for many of the people that I have worked with, who live with little or no ability to speak. I have found that using switches and alternative mouse devices like eyegaze for independent computer use, leisure and control of the environment can provide a person with control skills. These may be employed and developed to augment their spoken communication using a speech output device, just as you may have heard Professor Stephen Hawking use, for example.

*

When you are looking for technology to help you, it's important to find a company or an individual to work with you on a one-to-one basis, who will take the time to understand what it is that you need. It isn't just about the equipment.

As I am not affiliated with any one provider, I am able to provide a product agnostic service, giving you access to a mix of tools and ingredients that will help you to do what you are striving to do. It's a bespoke set-up that gives you the opportunity to trial and test the equipment to make sure that it is really right for you. People tell me that my intervention has changed their life for the better in so many ways.

*

Taking on new technology informs as much as it empowers. It enables people to see what is out there to help them, so that they can make informed choices about what they want to achieve and what their priorities are. The longer I spend with a user, the more innovations and developments we can make, as we learn – sometimes by accident and sometimes by design – what works for them.

Part 3

Hope for a Brighter Future

The Recovery Journey Never Really Ends, But There Are Better Days Ahead…

15 Funding Your Future

At some point, you will need to consider whether you may have a claim for compensation and the financial ramifications of your accident. Who should you approach about a claim, what does it involve and once you receive damages, how do you invest it to make sure it pays for the services you will need for the rest of your life.

Carolyn (Serious Injury Solicitor):

As a specialist solicitor at Irwin Mitchell, I work with adults and children who have sustained severe brain and/or spinal cord damage. The work that we do is very specialist and some of the cases we deal with – like Joe's – are large and complex. Essentially, our aim is always to put our client in the best possible position after their accident and make sure their quality of life is as good as it can be.

Injuries don't come much worse than Joe's and if you are reading this as someone who has gone through something similar – or as a friend or relative of someone who has – I'm sure you appreciate just how devastating it is. One of our main focusses at IM is to ensure that our clients have access to first class rehabilitation as soon as possible as it's rehabilitation and having the right support that will help to make our injured client as healthy, independent and happy as possible.

But where does the money come from to fund the rehabilitation packages and the compensation that the claimant now needs to fund the losses they have incurred and the services they now need?

In order to get compensation, you have to prove that somebody has done something wrong; another person has been negligent. Negligence consists of three things. The first is 'liability,' sometimes known as fault, which involves assessing whether the other person's behaviours and actions have fallen below a reasonable standard. The second element is known as "causation" i.e. did the accident cause your injuries and loss. This is usually straight forward but if someone already has a complicated medical history or

DOI: 10.4324/9781003430728-18

their own actions also contributed towards their injuries, "causation" may need to be investigated too. The third element is 'loss and damage' and involves looking at the extent of the injured person's injuries and the financial losses they will incur both now and in the future. If the claimant cannot establish all three things, there is no compensation.

Normally the burden is on the claimant, (the person bringing the claim) to prove that someone else (the defendant) was negligent. In Joe's case – as the claimant – it was our job to prove that the driver of the vehicle in which he was travelling was negligent.

Accidents happen in various ways e.g. on the roads, at work or tripping over something, and normally there is insurance in place somewhere along the line to cover the accident and any potential claims, but if there is no insurance we have to consider whether the person/organisation who caused the accident is financially worth suing. An exception to this relates to road traffic accidents. Car insurance is compulsory in the UK, and it is a criminal offence to drive a vehicle on the road if there is no insurance in place. Unfortunately, people don't always take insurance out and if the driver of an uninsured car is negligent, a claimant may, in certain circumstances, be able to bring a claim against a government body called the Motor Insurance Bureau.

Fortunately, there was insurance in Joe's case.

It can take time for both parties to investigate what actually happened in an accident and before the defendant confirms their position on liability. So where does that leave the claimant in terms of rehabilitation?

The early stages after an accident are incredibly traumatic for both clients and their families. Even as people are wrestling with huge life-or-death questions, there are still mortgages/rent and bills to be paid, and jobs and families to look after. So it is really important to try and get the injured person and their immediate family the help and support they need to get through this horrific time, something which I think Irwin Mitchell is very good at.

First, Irwin Mitchell has the advantage of having a wonderful group of Support and Rehab Coordinators, which includes therapists, nurses, teachers and social workers and it is their role to support our clients and help them through the strange and difficult world that they have now entered because of their or a loved one's injuries. Our Support & Rehabilitation Coordinators (SRCs) listen to and support our clients, they help signpost them to a number of organisations, for example, the NHS, social services, relevant charities or, if necessary, they will deal with these services direct. They can provide practical help and also liaise with employers and schools and help navigate clients through the very complicated world of benefits.

Second, our clients can have access to a financial health check carried out by our colleagues at Irwin Mitchell Asset Management (IMAM) as explained by John below. The injured person and family members will normally have to take time off work and the stress of worrying about your next mortgage payment or how your family are going to manage financially can be huge which is why IMAM offer a financial health check because in our view, in the months following the accident you should be concentrating on getting better, not worrying about money!

Third, if you were injured in a general accident e.g. road traffic accident, you may be able to get some help and rehabilitation under The Code of Rehabilitation. Claimants' solicitors – such as Irwin Mitchell – and defendant insurers can sign up to the Code, which encourages the parties to work together and agree a plan for the implementation of early rehabilitation. Basically, when we write to the defendant to tell them that our client is bringing a claim, we also ask them to agree to an immediate needs assessment (INA) under the Code of Rehabilitation. If the defendant agrees, a nominated person, normally a health professional, will assess the claimant and then write a report known as an INA, which makes recommendations for the immediate help and rehabilitation the claimant needs e.g. care/therapies/equipment and in some cases the setting up of a taxi account so the injured person can get to appointments etc. Once the INA is completed, the defendant insurer will then decide which if any of the recommendations they will fund. Some fund all, some fund some and some fund none! Unfortunately, as the Code is voluntary, there is little we can do if the defendant refuses to agree to an INA or later refuses to fund the recommendations made in the report.

Unfortunately, the Code of Rehabilitation doesn't apply to all claims so if the claimant's injuries were caused by say the NHS in a medical accident, you would not be able to benefit from the Code. Fortunately, at IM, all of our personal injury clients are able to access our SRCs and a financial health check which can really help.

If liability looks straight forward from the beginning, we can ask the defendant for an immediate interim payment in the early stages of the claim so that rehabilitation can be provided and money can be paid to help the client with their own financial commitments. If liability is more complicated, both parties will need to investigate the accident before interim payments are made for rehabilitation and the client as explained below.

Joe's Case:

Joe's family where initially supported by the Day One Trauma Charity and as one of their panel solicitors, his family asked if they could meet with us. I met with Joe's parents and his sister initially as it was very early days and Joe was still very poorly at that stage. When I did finally see him in person, we had a chat and I told him about what a claim involves, and he confirmed that he would like to instruct me. Over the years I have found that some clients want to leave everything up to you, some want their family to be involved and some, like Joe, want very much to be involved and to make their own decisions.

Shortly after meeting Joe I wrote to the defendant's solicitors, intimating the claim and setting out the catastrophic nature of Joe's injuries so they were in no doubt about how badly injured he was. An INA was requested and was later agreed. Whilst the Defendant solicitors were sympathetic to Joe's situation, this was a very high-value claim and it is their job to fully investigate every angle to protect their insurer client just like it is my job to protect my client's position. As a result, liability can take some time to resolve in the big catastrophic injury cases because very large sums of money are at stake, so the defendant is not going to admit liability until they have seen all available evidence and are completely satisfied that they are going to have to pay out. They will also look to see if there is any contributory negligence, see below. Both parties naturally need to see the police report and gather as much information as possible, so they know how strong their case is. For various reasons it took some time to get the police report in this case and there were also various other issues that had to be resolved e.g., which insurer was going to pick up the tab.

Eventually the defendant team confirmed that "primary" liability would not be an issue, after all cars don't just veer off the road, hit lampposts and flip over, but they reserved their position on what's known as contributory negligence which essentially means, did the injured person's own actions contribute to the accident circumstances or their injuries. Unfortunately, in Joe's case he wasn't wearing his seat belt at the time of the crash which impacted on the severity of his injuries and ultimately lead to his damages being reduced. In relation to seat belts, the extent of the reduction in your damages depends upon whether and to what extent the seat belt would have made a difference to your injuries. So if you would still have obtained the same injuries had you been wearing a seat belt there is no reduction as the outcome would have been the same. If you would have sustained less serve injuries, then you can generally lose up to 15% or so or your damages and if the seat belt would have prevented the injury altogether you can lose up to 25% of your damages. In high value cases, any reduction can have severe consequences as it eats into the money the injured person will need in order to pay for the huge amount of services and help they will now need for the rest of their life.

Due to the initial investigations into liability, it took some time to get an interim payment so that Joe could at last start to get the private rehabilitation he needed although he continued to have access to our SRCs. Once the insurer who ultimately paid the claim was satisfied about certain matters, it became much easier to get interim payments which really helped and meant that Joe could pay for things like private therapies, a case manager and a personal assistant was recruited who was in addition to his normal carers, see below. Joe also trialled and then bought assistive technology so that for the first time since his accident he could use his phone and computers by himself without having to have someone assist him which gave him back a huge degree of independence and much needed privacy. As time went on the interim payments allowed him to buy other equipment and he also purchased and adapted a house. I must acknowledge how helpful the defendants' solicitors and insurers were in this case once their initial investigations had taken place. They were certainly no push over and stood their ground on certain issues, but they were practical and sensible and assisted when they could. I also think Joe's determination and resilience helped and they seemed to respect the way he just tried to get on with everything and make a better life for himself despite the huge obstacles he faced every day.

Assessing the Value of a Claim:

Once liability has been established or we get to a position where we think we will win, we begin to look at quantum, which is the value of the case.

In order to value a case, we get experts to help us. In particular, we get medical experts, normally doctors at consultant level, to comment upon the injuries sustained, what the recovery is likely to be and what problems the client is likely to have in the short, medium, and long term. This is known as a long-term prognosis. If someone is catastrophically injured, it may not be possible for the medical experts to provide an opinion for some time. This can be because their injuries will take some time to settle down and/or they may need rehabilitation so that they can make as good a recovery as possible. Only when these things take place can the doctors normally try to work out what the injured person will be capable of in the future, e.g., work and what services they will now need for the rest of their life.

Depending upon how fiercely liability is fought, you can normally settle a catastrophic adult brain/spinal injury case or a child spinal case, from a quantum perspective, within two to three years. If your client is a brain-injured child though, it may be very different, and it could be a number of years before the case settles. How we cope as adults with such thing as organisation/planning is very much affected by the frontal lobes in our brains. These don't develop until our teenage years, and they continue to develop into our 20s. The doctors in those cases need to have a good idea about whether a child's frontal lobes have been affected by the accident and if that looks likely, you would not normally settle that case until the child is at least 16 and has completed their GCSEs and preferably between the ages of 18–21 or so when they have more life experience and you can see how they are coping.

In high value and particularly, catastrophic injury cases, we also get expert evidence from care experts, OT's (equipment/transport), Assistive Technology experts (IT/environmental controls), Therapists, (physio and speech and language) and accommodation experts on housing needs.

In Joe's case, there were 15 experts for him including liability and causation experts, numerous doctors and the non-medical experts mentioned above. The defence team had 15 experts too and there was also a joint expert appointed by both parties. The quantum evidence covered numerous things, e.g., Joe's extensive care needs, specialist equipment and transport, the future medical treatment he may need, therapies, housing even down to such things as the extra costs that Joe will now incur if he goes on holiday because he now needs a team of carers to go with him, all of whom have travel and accommodation costs which Joe has to pay for.

Before completing their reports, the experts will have access to various records including medical, employment, social services/ education and, if there is private rehabilitation package in place which is frequently the case, the records of the treating team. These documents can run into several thousands of pages and before they are sent to the experts (and the defence team) we have to scrutinise them to make sure they don't breach GDPR or contain legally privileged information and we also look to see if any of the entries helps our case or potentially damages our case as we cannot pick and choose what is disclosed. The process of dealing with the records is called "disclosure," and this is an ongoing issue throughout the claim.

During the life of the claim, we also prepare witness statements both for liability and quantum. In relation to quantum, the statements tend to be from family/friends, teachers/employers and the case manager who runs the post-accident private rehabilitation team. A statement from a family member will normally comment upon what the client was like before the accident, what their difficulties are now, how the accident has changed them and their lives and what help they need now etc. If the statement is from an employer, it will set out what the claimant did before their accident in terms of work, what they earned, what promotions they had already obtain and what promotions they may have had, had the accident not occurred and if there were any pre accident employment issues e.g. warnings etc. Joe ran his own building company at the time of the accident so we had to spend time looking at how his business would have grown and what his income was likely to have been over his working life had the accident not occurred.

The experts mentioned above consider the records and the witness statements and they also examine/assess the client and then prepare their reports. Once their reports are finalised the parties exchange the reports and then the experts for both sides meet in order to discuss their reports and see what, if anything, can be agreed. They then prepare a joint statement for the Court which sets out what has been agreed and what remains in issue.

Once the above has all been completed, the parties try to settle the case and if this cannot be done the matter will proceed to Trial where a Judge will then determine what the case is worth. Trials are expensive and can be very stressful for everyone involved so the parties are encouraged to negotiate a settlement if they can and most of the time that is exactly what happens.

At the beginning of this chapter, I talked about rehabilitation and how important that is and from Irwin Mitchell's perspective it really is crucial and core to everything we do. If you are seriously injured you want to be able to pay for the care, therapies, equipment, transport and housing you now need but as with us all, what you really want is a decent quality of life and to be happy. Having compensations means you can pay for the services you need and it gives you choices but if you cannot do anything for yourself or you are in pain constantly, etc., the money is unlikely to make you happy. Having access to good rehabilitation so that you become stronger, more independent and healthier is crucial.

Here at IM, we keep a close eye on our client's rehabilitation and how it progresses as does the defendant because they want to make sure it is costs effective and working just as much as we do.

We also have to support the injured person and their family through the process as it can be very difficult to suddenly have a large care or treating team in your home and at first the lack of privacy and disruption to family this causes can be difficult. Families can struggle with this in the beginning but normally things bed down quickly and everyone sees just how helpful and important the support is.

Each rehab and care team is tailored to suit the client's need. As you will have read in other paragraphs, Joe wasn't going to let being a ventilated quadriplegic stop him and from early on he was determined to get on with things and carve a new future for himself. He did some work, threw himself into studying, set up a charity and bought and adapted a house! As a ventilated quadriplegic with numerous health issues each of these things was no easy feat let alone doing all four together. Being paralysed from the neck down means that Joe cannot do much for himself so it was important for Joe to have assistive technology and also a personal assistant in addition to his carers who could support him with everything he was doing and this was costed for within his claim.

If a client has a brain injury, we need to know the extent of the damage and also whether the client is capable of managing the litigation (claim) themselves and also their financial affairs.

In relation to managing the litigation, if someone is not capable of managing the claim themselves or, if they are a child/young person under the age of 18, a litigation friend has to be appointed to deal with the claim on their behalf. This is often a family member, partner, or friend and if no one is available to take on this role the Official Solicitor is approached to see if they will act in that capacity.

In relation to financial affairs, if an adult is not capable of managing these any compensation, they receive will be paid into the Court of Protection which is part of the Court structure in England and Wales. The Court administer the client's money via a 'Deputy' who liaises between the injured person and the Court of Protection in relation to budget, investments and anything that the injured person may need. There are costs implications to being in the Court of Protection but these costs are claimed in the claim as well as it is normally an extra expense caused by the accident.

Whilst the claim is ongoing, we need to know about how any interim payments are being spent and on what so that we can plan and budget accordingly and make sure the client has enough money to pay for the services they need now e.g., therapies. This is regardless of whether the client can manage their finances or not.

Choosing a Solicitor:

Clients only get one shot at getting the compensation they need to pay for a lifetime of losses and services, so it is very important to make sure you chose a solicitor with the right experience who knows about catastrophic injuries, rehabilitation and things like the Court of Protection. I sometimes have to interview solicitors for jobs at Irwin Mitchell and there are some questions I often put to the candidate because it tells me straight away how much experience they have in brain and spinal cord work. These questions are just as valid for any client, or a member of their family, looking to appoint a solicitor for someone with a catastrophic injury like Joe's and they are:

- How many brain/spinal cases have you handled?
- What was your highest settlement?
- How many large rehabilitation packages have you put in place and what did the biggest ones involve?
- What do you know about the Court of Protection and how many of your clients are in the Court of Protection (for brain injury cases)?
- How many houses have you bought for clients with physical difficulties?

If you have appointed a solicitor and are concerned that things are not progressing, you are not getting interim payments and the rehabilitation you need, or the service you are generally getting is poor then you can change solicitors and we certainly offer a second opinion here at IM.

Related charities are also a good way of trying to find suitable solicitors. I mentioned Day One earlier, which operates in the major trauma centres in Leeds, Aintree, and at James Cook. They have a ward case worker who can arrange for patients to speak to a solicitor from their specially selected panel of firms. There are also charities like Headway for brain injury, and the Spinal Injuries Association, as well as Joe's own charity, Quad-Rebuild. You will find a full list of charities and other helpful resources at the back of the book.

After settlement, it is very important to invest your money in an appropriate way as the money will have to last for your lifetime and pay for what you need. Having good advice from people who understand what you need to pay for in life is crucial and John is going to talk about that later on.

Looking to the Future:

Over the course of nearly 30 years, I've worked with some truly inspirational clients who have done phenomenally well after catastrophic injures and Joe is certainly one of those clients. He really has been inspirational and to watch him go from strength to strength and be so determined not just to create a positive life for himself but also try to help others via his charity is very humbling and as with other clients it tends to put my own moans and groans into perspective. He's a character, totally driven, utterly frustrating at times but kind, funny, hardworking with fierce determination and as I say and as I think the defendants saw, he's truly inspirational. It has been a pleasure to act for him.

John (Chartered Financial Planner at IM Asset Management Limited):

As Carolyn says, the way in which we manage our clients' money is designed to make a real difference, and that's what makes this job so rewarding.

Our advice is holistic. This involves having a good understanding of a person's care needs, and considering all the things they might need money for – both now and in the future – including property purchase, adaptations, vehicles, specialist equipment etc. It's about making sure that clients like Joe have the right consideration of their many and complex needs over the long term.

I often meet clients before their case is settled. The likelihood is that they will be going through a really tough time at that stage. Like Joe, many of our clients have had a catastrophic injury and their world has been turned upside down. When people have had a significant, life-changing injury their focus is understandably going to be on other non-financial things. They may be rebuilding their lives, looking after kids, or just trying to get back to some sort of normality.

As a result of an accident, an individual may have lost their job and be in financial difficulty. They often have money worries. A Financial Questionnaire is completed with a client to get a good understanding of their current financial position, and this can sometimes identify shortfalls. Is it possible to reduce expenditure? Cancelling subscriptions, reducing hidden expenditure, and making financial savings are not necessarily going to be top of anyone's list of priorities at that stage in their recovery. However, discussing budgets and creating a more structured approach to managing their finances can reduce stress and develop better spending habits. Thus, allowing a client to focus on the more important things in their life.

Having an improved understanding of financial planning also reduces the potential of an individual being overwhelmed when their Personal Injury claim finally settles as managing a large financial settlement can be daunting.

If you are embarking on this process yourself – or you're helping somebody who is – there are several factors to consider when choosing who you want to work with. Perhaps the biggest factor is – who do you trust?

You need to establish a strong, trusting relationship with your advisor. This person will get to know you over a long period of time. They will come to your house every year to update you on your investment portfolio. And there will inevitably be years when they deliver less favourable news. There will be times when investment portfolios don't perform as well. For example, rising inflation – as we have at the time of writing – can have a big impact on the markets. So that personal connection and that trust are really important factors in choosing who you want to work with.

I visited Joe at home a few times to start to build that relationship. I explained to Joe, and his fellow Trustee, Liam, how we would work with him and help him manage his money. Initially we discussed Joe's plans and how his monies could be structured to meet his needs. Joe was given some examples of suitable savings accounts for Trusts and we explored longer term investments. Past performance, which isn't a guarantee to the future, along with suitable tax planning and charges were discussed to give Joe an insight of how we help clients. After a few meetings the advice became more bespoke to Joe, establishing more accurately his financial requirements and what level of risk he was comfortable with before formalising a plan.

Making the Right Decisions for Your Financial Future:
I would go through a similar process with you...

With your settlement assured we would discuss your plans. It's important that we dig a bit deeper and get a good understanding of your needs, both now and in the long term.

This involves a review of your current financial position, looking at monthly income and expenditure, any planned capital expenditure you may have and how much should be held in cash to cover these short-term needs. We would also discuss how much should be securely held in cash for contingency. From experience, contingency planning is so important.

You may find that you have different financial needs at the start of the process. It's quite understandable that many of our clients want to treat themselves when a settlement comes through. They have been through so much that they may want to take an expensive holiday or treat themselves to something in the first year or two.

Some of your settlement may be required for buying a house or making suitable adaptations to an existing house. Due to the pandemic, we have seen adaptations costing more than initially planned, therefore highlighting the importance of a suitable contingency fund. There may be occasions when I need to present another point of view to you – if something is not affordable, or if it might be better to wait before purchasing something – I'll lay out the pros and cons for you. Once we know how much money you may need for planned capital expenditure, such as property purchase, adaptations, equipment, or other necessity, we would then discuss longer term investments. This gives me a clear picture of how much is affordable for you to invest. I would explain how investments work, explore different types of investments, assess your attitude to risk and discuss suitable tax planning solutions. It can take several meetings to assess all your requirements and put a tailored action plan in place. We don't rush into investing monies.

I often find that, after a year or two, clients develop a much closer and deeper understanding of their ongoing financial requirements, and may voluntarily reduce their spending, or flex their investment as existing investments change and develop. You may well find that you need to see less and less of me throughout the year when you feel better equipped to oversee your financial future.

I aim to give clients ongoing financial independence. Together, we will make sound investments without taking any unnecessary risks. Like Joe, you may have a personal injury trust (managed by Trustees), and I'll help you explore their legalities and benefits, and explain how it will be administered in your case.

Working with Joe:

Right from the start, I could see that Joe was a wonderful character. When he decided he wanted to work with us, I began by getting an understanding of the kind of structure he needed to have in place, making sure he had the right amount of money in the right place that will be accessible at the right time so that he can crack on with his life and pay for what he needs to whilst also being able to do things that are important to him.

After a few meetings we were able to finalise our bespoke advice for Joe. The objective of our plan is to ensure that Joe can pay for the services he needs and be financially comfortable throughout his lifetime. We now have investments growing for him that will be accessed to top up his cash accounts whenever he needs them.

I enjoy working with Joe. He's a hundred-miles-an-hour chap! He contacts me regularly to ask what I think of his plans, such as potential further property purchases. One of the reasons for leaving a suitable contingency fund at the outset was so that he could take some overseas holidays, as going on holiday was one of his great passions before the accident.

Joe is a good example of how capital expenditure changes as time goes on. We expected that Joe might want to use some of his settlement in the early days. He had been though a horrific time in his life. He also had immediate pressing needs for a new property and equipment. The holidays were important too. So we planned for all of that, but with the expectation that his expenditure would slow down as the years went on.

We're always here for our clients whenever they need us; sometimes that's to answer questions about their portfolios, sometimes it's just for reassurance. Most of our clients are clients because they've had an injury. They're not experienced investors. They weren't expecting to be working with a financial planner, and they won't necessarily know what to expect. They may not come from a wealthy background. The money they have, and the settlement they're getting are critically important. They can watch the news and see markets fluctuating and panic. So, of course, I'm here if they ring up in a panic and say, "John, what's going to happen to my money?!"

The world of personal injury claims is a very different place to other branches of financial planning. It's incredibly rewarding to work with people like Joe to help them ensure their financial future is positive so they can focus on what they want to achieve.

16 Care and Support

Joe's team admits that while their roles bring many unexpected challenges, it is a mutually rewarding experience. Here, they talk about the day-to-day realities of the work they do.

Working with Joe is all about learning how we overcome challenges, and the more we learn, the more Joe wants to feed back into the community of people who will be facing similar issues to him.

Hayley (PA):

Right from the start, I could see that Joe was (and remains) very driven. I found him honest and outspoken too; passionate about a lot of things, and this all helps keep him going. Joe's will and his self-belief are incredibly strong, and they have allowed him to achieve so much, but I know it has been frustrating for him at times not to be able to do everything that he wants to do as easily as other people can. He recognised that he needed help with so many of the practical elements of his life, so I help him achieve the things he wants to achieve.

I appreciate that Joe has had to put a lot of trust and faith in me. And Joe has said that sometimes, that has been what he has really struggled with. He's gone from being really independent to having to rely on other people, and trust in the fact that they're doing what they're supposed to be doing for him. In a way he has no choice but to rely on other people to be able to get things done, and I think that he has been learning to accept that too. Joe has had to deal with a lot of different people having access to his life – and his personal life – in ways he wouldn't have expected. And that can feel quite invasive, so it has been helpful for me to deal with some of that for him.

The work that I do – and Joe's carers do – is incredibly diverse. As well as overseeing his healthcare, he wanted me to assist him and his sister in running his business, and setting up his charity.

DOI: 10.4324/9781003430728-19

Really, I'm more of a lifestyle PA. I look after everything, from overseeing the back and forth of information with solicitors relating to his litigation case, to liaising with the care team about his care package, and even personal things – in relation to family events, and helping him keep on top of all the developments with his house build.

In the nicest possible way, I'm a bit like damage control! I'm like a little buffer, so if Joe is struggling, his family can talk to me. I can tell them, honestly, how Joe is doing, and that's just easier for Joe. Not because he doesn't want to speak to them, but because sometimes, he knows he can't give people what they want to hear. In a way, it's a bit like having an extension to my own family.

One of the things that we've found helpful – that might also help you, if you're adjusting to a changed life after an accident like Joe had – is simplifying the day-to-day. Joe's care package encompasses so much; it's not just clinical, it's keeping his house together and so many little day-to-day things, from shopping to taxing his car. I can help with all these things as required, so that if Joe is having a difficult day and requires more direct care from his team, I can step in and look after things and keep his life admin ticking over.

Essentially, I have an overarching perspective over each element of his life, and I am usually the first point of contact, whether it's family calling, or the care team, or Joe himself, calling for some sort of support. In meetings I represent Joe quite a lot. He may not have the time or the energy to devote to all of those things, so I am effectively his voice. Taking some of these things off Joe's shoulders allows him to go to work and focus on his job, without having to worry about his care package, or any of the hundreds of things that would be very onerous for him. If there is someone in your life that can help you by administering some of these things for you – it doesn't have to be a PA – I think that can be very helpful.

Working with Joe is all about learning how we overcome challenges, and the more we learn, the more Joe wants to feed back into the community of people who will be facing similar issues to him. He does appreciate that he's lucky to have a PA when so many people don't. We know there are too many people, like him – who want to start again, and who want to achieve things – who don't have the same resource. His experiences have taught him so much that he wants to extend a helping hand to as many others as he can. We have to remember that people's injuries can be so physically debilitating; they may not be able to write or contact someone without assistance; there are so many things that most of us take for granted that can be really taxing for somebody. Even signing documents – you'd think that would be paperless, but it often isn't – can be beyond somebody's altered capability. He's working hard on finding ways to help people with issues like this through the Quad-Rebuild charity. And one of the biggest benefits of working with Joe is that it's been so nice to help him push his charity forwards, and work towards achieving some of his dreams. I think you will find that too if you are helping somebody.

The role has its own challenges, and no two days are the same. It can obviously be impacted by Joe's health, and it can be hard to adjust if he is feeling bad. Joe is incredibly strong, but inevitably, his mood can dip, and it can be tough to stay positive and help him through that. But I do know now that I'm not there to fix every problem; sometimes I just need to listen. There will be times when Joe needs to offload, and I can help him with that, but it's all about judging the mood of the day. There will be times when we need to take a step back, and there will be other times when we just need to crack on with some of the jobs we have to do that day. And if you're helping someone, you will find that fine line, together.

One thing I have learned from being with Joe is that the sooner you're able to treat each other without feeling like you're walking on eggshells, the better it will be. There aren't any airs and graces between us – not many PAs go into their office and need to scratch their boss's nose, or have to take action if he or she is struggling to breathe.

So this really has been a totally new working environment for me as a PA, and I think the same goes for care staff; this job isn't like many other care roles...

Gez (Carer):

That's true. It was quite a challenge at first. I was working through my psychology degree when I was given the opportunity to support Joe, and learn more about care work. My degree studies only took me so far; I didn't have any experience of catheters or tracheostomies, so that was quite daunting. Joe's case is very complex; it's not like a normal care home job. There is always a lot to do, so everyone chips in and helps out. As a result, I found that I was learning on the job very quickly, but you are always aware of the importance of the care you're providing, and how essential the work you're doing is.

Hayley (PA):

Emotionally, this can be a hard job. If I ever had any doubts about my suitability for the role it was because in the early days, I didn't quite appreciate the full extent of Joe's condition. It was hard seeing everything that he had to endure, and it was eye-opening seeing what needed to happen just to keep him alive.

Gez (Carer):

There were some challenging moments with Joe; his tracheostomy blocked, and he couldn't breathe, so we had to run through a list of procedures, one by one, in an effort to get him breathing, quickly. There was a time when Joe's blood pressure shot up to 220 and we called an ambulance. But they just weren't used to dealing with somebody like Joe with such complex needs, and in that circumstance, the carer almost becomes an advocate. The career has to know everything about the person they're caring for so that they can assist the medical staff.

It can be quite frustrating for Joe if the hospital medical staff are doing things their way and that didn't correspond with his (and our) understanding of how things should be done for him. It's really important that continuity of care remains in place. So, for as long as Joe was in hospital, we would always go in and ensure that his care was continuing in the right way.

Hayley (PA):

I think the jobs of PA and carer for somebody in Joe's position do require different skillsets, and that's one reason why, if you or a loved one are looking for a PA or care support, it's worth taking the time to try and find people you really feel you can work with.

As a PA, I can tell you that it's not like any other admin role with a clear picture of what you're going to be doing day by day. In theory, I do have contracted hours of work, but the nature of this job is that I'm available to help Joe beyond that too. Practically, I know that if Joe is in hospital for a few days, then I still need to keep everything ticking along in his absence. It doesn't all stop! There is always a lot going on, and as his main point of contact, I have to make sure that by the time he returns, he can pick up life, work, and everything else.

It's important for Joe to have the security of knowing that there's always someone there looking out for him, and standing by to help him. That has been a learning curve for us both. Joe is learning to become a boss of managing his own lifestyle, and that's hard. Most of us have the luxury of thinking, *I want to do that*, and then we do it. But it doesn't work like that for Joe. He had to learn to accept our role in helping him do what he wants to do.

Gez (Carer):

It's true, this really isn't just another nine-to-five job. It can go way beyond the job description, and you have to be fully invested in it. There weren't any typical days with Joe!

Joe was almost always awake quite early. We would start by getting him ready for the day and then be ready for anything and everything, from assisting him with his work to preparing meals, to supporting him with his university work. Basically, it could be anything that Joe would otherwise have been able to do on his own before the accident. It could be anything as seemingly straightforward as checking a weather app or scrolling through Instagram, or putting a picture on social media. As Haley said, it was part of our jobs to help him achieve those things that he could no longer achieve on his own.

Joe uses an eyegaze computer, but with so much that he wanted to achieve each and every day, he usually found that he could do more by getting us to help him with as many of his projects as possible. While he can do a number of those things himself, it uses up a lot of energy; it really can leave him feeling quite drained. So, it makes more sense to let us deal with as many of those things as possible.

Hayley (PA):

Even though no two days are ever the same, there are certain set roles that I need to work on each week, irrespective of whatever else is happening. I oversee a lot of his communications, and his personal finances. Joe likes to look at developing land and properties, and I help him with researching costs – outgoings of material and contractor payments – plus keeping on top of the spreadsheets. The charity is a big focus for Joe. I helped him get the charity number and go through the application process with the trustees.

I have monthly meetings with his care manager. Because I can see how the process works on both sides of the equation, I provide a bit of objectivity and insight into any issues that may have arisen. In spite of his strength of character and his determination, Joe can be vulnerable, so it's important that we're always looking at the bigger picture to ensure Joe gets the support and care he needs at all times.

If Joe is going on holiday, I sort out the travel arrangements and bookings, and carry out all the necessary risk assessments for each destination. I will also ensure he has all the necessary medical equipment, and organise the insurance. His care team obviously need to travel with him, so booking a weekend away is quite a big deal. There will be four carers on every day, so it is a bit like preparing a small army!

Joe is a busy guy; he does nearly everything that he wants to do, so looking after his calendar is important, and I make sure that Joe gets all the notifications for meetings and phone calls via Alexa, so that he never misses anything.

Gez (Carer):

He almost always had a million things going on in his life; more things than most people who have full mobility actually. As carers, we were there to help him in doing as many of those things as were practical.

Hayley (PA):

Joe is almost always on the go, always thinking and planning, and working on something. There are certainly times when I'm flagging at the end of the day and he is still going strong, and I have to tell him I'm done for the day! There's usually a lot of banter between us, and he likes that. He appreciates working with people who see him for who he is. And if you're in the position of caring for someone or providing a little bit of assistance, don't be too hard on yourself if it takes you a little while to find your feet with that person. If you knew them before, it might take a while to adjust to the fact that they have changed, but you will come to see the ways in which they're still the same person underneath. It's alright to allow yourself some time to take that on board.

I hadn't known Joe before, but it took me a bit of time to get comfortable in that environment. In the early days, I jumped any time one of his machines bleeped and wondered if he was okay. And he'd have to tell me I'm fine, stop asking. It took a lot of learning, but we've got comfortable with each other over time, and we've learned to be ourselves with each other. I think that's really important. He doesn't want me to sugar-coat things, and he's quite prepared for us to clash over certain things, but he appreciates my honesty.

Gez (Carer):

As in any close working relationship it is almost inevitable that there will be occasional clashes. But don't worry, your carer will have a thick skin; they will be resilient. And, of course, you are allowed to be angry. You and your carers will work out how to deal with that anger or unhappiness in a way that works for you. From my own experience, there were times when Joe's anger got the better of him, and in those situations, it was sometimes better to just walk away from the situation and take a few minutes to just calm down.

Michaela (Joe's Sister):

We don't mollycoddle him. Not at all. We just treat him like Joe, and I think that's really important. Now, if he's being rude, we'll tell him straight. We'll argue back with him if we need to. He might not like it, but that's part and parcel of being in a family.

You have to be able to let them find their own ways of objecting/ fighting back too. When Joe doesn't want to speak to us, he can't get up and walk away, or wave us away. Instead, he shuts his eyes. So that's his way of saying I'm not speaking to you about this. We have to give him a little bit of time to think about things.

He'll say it to his carers sometimes too. There will be times when things just get to much for him, and he'll have to ask them to give him some space and leave him alone for a little bit. And again, I think it's really important that someone has the power to say that. They need to be able to go on expressing their wishes with as much power as before. Joe is looked after night and day, so he has no private time, and he needs that.

Hayley (PA):

By now at least, I think he knows that there are times when he can at least switch off, knowing that everything that needs to be done is being taken care of for him, without him needing to check up one every last little thing. It's amazing how much knowing that the little things are being taken care of can help you take care of the bigger things. And with so many other things going on in his life, he needed that, he needed a PA or someone to be that go-to-person and give him that support. There isn't much that can stop Joe now, and if there's a way around any problem, we'll find it.

Gez (Carer):

It isn't always easy to switch off from this kind of work. After spending so much time together and with members of Joe's family, we do start to feel like a part of an extended family. Certainly, Joe's dad was like a grandad to me in the time I was there. And I was full of respect and admiration for the support they give to Joe. They have had so much to deal with, and they have all managed to accept and come to terms with everything that has happened.

Hayley (PA):

Switching off is really critical for all of us. Of course, I am absolutely invested in Joe's life. I'm looking after so many of his affairs, and working with him to make some of the big decisions around his care, or his legal case, or his charity and going on those journeys with him that it's impossible not to be a part of his life and his family.

Joe will usually tell me to go home on Friday and switch off it from it all. But it isn't always that simple. If Joe goes into hospital at one in the morning, I'm his point of contact, and I'll be notified. As well as hoping that everything is going to be alright, I'll switch straight back into work mode and start thinking through what I'll need to do the next day to keep his affairs running smoothly in his absence.

So, it can feel hard to detach from it all sometimes, and I do urge you to find ways of leaving the work behind at the end of the day. It's important for you to know your boundaries so you can switch off as far as possible.

Gez (Carer):

I think the single most important thing for new carers is to try not to take anything too personally. You might hear foul language, you might feel that frustration, you might see shouting and anger; but you need to remember that none of it is your fault. And more importantly, you need to accept that this person's life has changed in every single way. Sometimes you'll need to take a step back and just settle yourself. Deep down that person respects and appreciates everything you do for them. Maybe they won't thank you for every little thing, but how can they? How can they possibly thank you for all of those little things you do? It would take forever.

I knew Joe was grateful. I knew that he felt the pressure of having to rely on other people to help him. And I know for sure that as long as there is mutual respect and friendship the relationship between a person and a carer will work. Show respect and your life as a carer will always be a successful one.

Michaela (Joe's Sister):

We all know there are going to be times when Joe gets frustrated. It was tough when he had to move hospitals, and when he was waiting to move into his adapted house. Maybe your family will be facing difficult anniversaries, or events that you can't enjoy in the same way, so I think it helps to plan for as many of these things as you can. Knowing that things are – or will be – difficult just helps you to understand, even if it's only a little bit, why Joe gets angry or frustrated. And we're there for him.

Gez (Carer):

With my interest in psychology, I was very invested in supporting Joe in terms of the care he required, but also in providing the emotional support he needed too. When we first met, he was going through a particularly tough time after his relationship had ended. It was very difficult for him, and there was nothing that anyone could do to take that pain away. That is made all the more difficult because there are times when you just want to give someone a hug, and that isn't really possible for Joe.

You have to accept that you can't say the same sorts of things to someone in that position that you might be able to say to a friend. It is so hard to see somebody going through that and not being able to help. We all know that in these situations, time is the only healer, but that doesn't help someone in the very raw stage of their grieving journey.

Inevitably, there were days when Joe was feeling the full extent of that sadness, and days when he was frustrated and angry. I think it's fair to say that everyone in that environment was in tears at some point; everyone felt their own frustration at not being able to do more.

Hayley (PA):

I think counselling has really helped Joe. It isn't just the physical side of things that needs to be addressed, it is the mental and wellbeing side of things. Having that kind of support can be so helpful. I know that, in the early days of his recovery, there were times when Joe felt incredibly vulnerable, and alone. Now, of course, Joe is never alone and that's a blessing and a curse. I know that he can sometimes feel lonely, but at other times, because he has 24-hour care, he feels like he can't have a moment to himself. We all know how important it is to have a few moments to ourselves, and he can't have that. But also, so much of his life, after the accident, has had to be focussed on the physical side, and it's hard to devote yourself to just concentrating on dealing with the physical impact, when you have suffered so much mentally too. So counselling is a really vital part of anyone's recovery process – and that goes for family members and friends too.

There are support groups out there; even just having something to distract you from the day-to-day, and having the chance to interact with other people and learn from their experiences can be really helpful. Joe has certainly made sure that he has kept taking trips and excursions, and there are charities that can help to support those kinds of adventures, such as his charity, Quad-Rebuild.

Gez (Carer):

You may even develop a good and potentially lasting friendship with your carer. Generally, a carer will work long shifts in your home. To your carer, it can almost feel like a second home. Joe really did become a friend to me, and even though we don't work together anymore, I will continue to keep in touch with him.

I was able to talk to Joe about his Masters studies, and talk to him about psychology. And having made those kinds of connections, it is sad to bring a professional relationship to an end. I think it really does help to be able to build up a friendship. It can be very obvious in a job like that if a career isn't really engaged with the work, or with the person they are caring for. They are the people that find it most difficult to be there. Even in my relatively short time with Joe I saw people come and go, and in almost every case, the people who left the quickest were the ones who didn't strike up any kind of bond with Joe.

That's not just important for them, it's important for him too. The person being cared for needs to be able to trust the people who are caring for them. It isn't just about the quality of the care they offer, it is about the courtesy and respect of getting to know that person. Joe was particularly keen to get to know every single carer. That's where a relationship built on trust begins. And that's where the roots of understanding begin too; being able to understand and even anticipate the needs of the person you're caring for makes the job of caring so much easier.

Hayley (PA):

I think that my work with Joe has helped him regain some of the trust that I think he'd lost from engaging with PAs in the early days after his accident, which did not go so well. I think at that time, he perhaps wasn't ready to go with quite as many of his plans, and it must have felt as if he was paying them for doing very little.

I know money is a barrier for some of the technology that Joe has used, or for hiring a full-time PA, but there are still things that are accessible which I think can really help everyone in this situation. But if you can't get a PA, there are virtual PAs out there who can really help you too! You can use their services for a few hours, or invest in a bank of time for specific tasks.

Gez (Carer):

Carers and PAs don't just get involved in helping you; they help your family too. After all, it's important to look after everyone who is involved. It's a much bigger job than I ever imagined; your carers are there to make your whole life easier and to do those things that you can no longer do.

Having a care team may sound challenging, it may sound like an imposition to have people you don't know coming into your home. But do be reassured that those people will do the very best job they can to support you or your loved one. If you have been in the position of looking after someone, they will help take some of the pressure off you so that you can achieve what you want to achieve, it is also important to understand the barriers when entering someone's home and respecting their wishes regarding what you can and cannot do.

Hayley (PA):

> Joe's own experience has also shown that it's never too late to learn new skills. Joe was a stonemason; he used his hands in his work and he was so good at what he did. It must have been a huge blow when that was taken away from him, but he looked for something else, and he found his university course. All sorts of things are out there and accessible to help you invest in the things you love, or in entirely new things.
>
> There are times when Joe feels lucky; he has his mind and the capability to do so much of what he wants to do. He feels as if everything that has happened has given him the opportunity to invest in his charity and help others.

Gez (Carer):

> I saw a massive change in Joe's mental state. It was amazing to see him become so much more positive – and so much more accepting – as time went on. By the time I left, he clearly had so much more to look forward to in his life. The biggest shift is that he now considers himself quite lucky and quite privileged in some ways to be able to pursue so many of the things he wants to pursue. He doesn't dwell on the fact that he can't move, he looks at the positives: his house, his charity, and the possibilities for his future developments, utilising his construction knowledge. I saw a huge improvement in his mental state, the person he was when I started working with him is not the person he is today.
>
> As for me, I want to go on to do a PhD in psychology and go into therapy. This job has really taught me a lot about myself and about where my future lies; I've certainly grown into a much more patient person. Working with Joe has shown me that I would like to work in hospital in the role of the therapist who goes to talks to people like Joe who have just suffered a massive trauma.

17 Letting Go and Moving On

When you come to accept that everything is different, and when you let go of what you have lost, you can finally start to forge a new life for yourself. It could even be a better life...

> *I feel energised and passionate about the future... I have been given an opportunity to help so many other people. I want to be able to look back when I'm older and be satisfied with my achievements.*

Joe:

Your life will never be the same again. That maybe a scary thought, but it can be liberating too.

Andy (Mentor Support):

I know what Joe means. After my accident, I tried to return to my previous job in mechanical engineering, that's what I wanted to do. But I wasn't able to reach the level of work I expected of myself, and I knew then that I had to try other things. And when I did, my world started to open up again.

Joe:

Wherever your new path takes you, you are going to have to come to terms with more than the injury. The hard truth is that the injury is just the start. You will have to accept the ways in which it is going to affect your entire life.

When I was starting all over again without some of the things that made me who I am, there were times when I just wanted to give in. There were times when I felt selfish, when I didn't think about my friends and family, and I just wanted to give in to the depression.

As well as my injury and loss of independence, I was grieving for the gradual loss of the business I had built from nothing, the loss of my relationship with the woman I loved, and the loss of my craft – stone carving.

DOI: 10.4324/9781003430728-20

It isn't easy, but you have to learn how to redirect your thoughts, feelings, and emotions to let go of things of value to you. Stone carving had defined me from a young age.

Michaela (Joe's Sister):

Joe used to work with his dad on all sorts of building projects from as young as five. He learnt stone masonry to a really high standard, and as you've heard, he won competitions for it. It was a massive part of his life, and of his identity. Coming to terms with losing something so important to him was really tough to deal with.

Joe:

I used to be able to lose myself in stone carving for hours on end. I just went into that focussed space and loved it. Whatever else was happening in my life, I knew I could let it all slip away when I was carving. I think everyone needs something like that in their life, something that takes them out of themselves. Accepting that I was not going to be able to do it anymore was one of the hardest things I have had to overcome.

I got locked in anger at times. I kept beating myself up about what had happened. In short, I just couldn't accept it for a very long time. And as long as I couldn't accept it, I couldn't move forwards.

Ross (Joe's Friend):

It wasn't just the horror of the injury, it was everything that he lost along with it. His job, his passion for stone carving, his girlfriend... How do you cope with losses like that?

Joe:

What I have learned from working with psychologists, and what I have come to understand for myself is that the dark times are a natural part of coming to terms with what has happened. Without grieving, or expressing your anger, you can't move on properly. You have to recognise your loss or your impediment and be honest about your struggles, whether that takes you a few months or a few years.

Like any other sort of grief, it is a process, just like losing a parent, or losing a partner. At the time, it is catastrophic, and overcoming it takes time. You need to allow yourself that time to grieve. Don't be too hard on yourself...

Michaela (Joe's Sister):

... And don't give up hope. Always believe in yourself (or your loved one) and in an ability to move past what has happened, but accept that it will take time. And accept that that there will be dark times, while knowing that as a family, or a couple, or as friends, you can come through them.

Joe:

What has happened to you is a traumatic injury; you need to be able to confront the feelings it brings out, and address the anger and grief that feel like they could overwhelm you. Your instinct might be to hide the unpleasant feelings, or try to pretend that you can move past them, but you can't. You can't change what has happened, and you can't undo it, no matter how hard you might wish it.

You have to be ready to accept and forgive. It was only when I was ready to accept that life would never be like it had been, and that the rest of my life wasn't going to turn out how I had planned, that I could forgive myself for my part in what had happened, and get some closure on it.

Until you are ready and able to do that, you will be stuck. You won't move forwards. The big message is that the longer it takes, the more of your life you're going to waste. I learned that the hard way.

Barry (Joe's Friend):

Joe was much too proud to let himself be beaten by his injury and its impact. And he was never one for taking sympathy very easily. If I tried to say how much I admired him for coping with it all, or how impressed everyone was with what he was achieving, he'd cut me off. "You'd do the same. Don't try and make me different from anybody else."

Joe didn't want people to look at him and feel sorry for him. He wanted them to look at him and say, 'That's Joe English, he's a great guy, or a great craftsman or whatever.' And it must have been difficult for him to have to adjust to a world in which people weren't going to say, "Joe's a great stonemason" any more...

Joe:

On the face of it, your hobbies, interests, and passions might not seem so important in the early days of your recovery when everything is focussed on surviving and talking the first steps towards recovery. But don't underestimate how important these things are to your sense of self, particularly as you progress through your recovery.

You have to find a way to deal with the loss of the things you love, and find new ways of embracing those things. One of the things I have learned to do is, instead of carving the stone myself, has been to appreciate the work and artistry in a fine piece of carving. Before, when I lost myself in it, I could be a bit reclusive, but I've found that now, it is a less lonely pursuit. I enjoy appreciating carving with others. And I have started researching different methods and architectural techniques, so I have a wider, more open appreciation of the art. I can appreciate the beauty of stone carving, and look at my craft in a completely different way.

Kate (Joe's Friend):

I used to get Joe to look at people who'd had similar accidents to him to see what they had achieved. And it would inspire him to try and achieve some of those things too. There are painters who have learned to paint with their mouth after surviving a paralysing accident.

Joe:

Not everything can be substituted by something else, but so many things can be. If you like cooking, perhaps you can discuss recipes with a friend or partner and then let them cook under your direction. Try and find some way – your way – of enjoying those things again. I didn't have to abandon my love of stone carving just because I couldn't physically do it anymore. Now, I truly love to see how a piece of stone is created, and tooled and moulded.

I always liked doing things in my own way, and now I can see that I was actually a little bit close-minded, and insular in my passions. But now, with a different take on things, I can appreciate stone masonry so much more.

Andy (Mentor Support):

I went through a similar process after my accident. I returned to education and got more qualifications. I started playing all sorts of sports, and embarked on further studies. In time, I learned to take any and every chance I got to do new things, and to travel.

Joe:

Not everyone has a clear idea of where they want to take their lives, and I think it's important to take as much help and support as you can get. Peer-level support from people who have experienced some of what you might be going through is really valuable.

My Quad-Rebuild charity is designed to help people cope with, adjust to, and overcome the constraints that bind so many of us after injury. It can be hard to know what we want in our lives when we don't know what help and support is out there to help us achieve those things. Anyone out there that needs help, guidance, and support can access it through our charity. We are here to help you find the path you want to take. Whether that is to help you feel more independent, or to give you the support you need to plan an overseas trip, or access training. Our charity is like no other, we don't put restrictions in place, we are here to offer a bespoke service to each and every client, there are no limitations to how we can help you in your life.

Life isn't about achieving as much as you can, it's about creating the life that works for you. And that's what each one of us, no matter the level or severity of our injury – should be entitled to do.

You don't have to do it alone. Help is out there.

Andy (Mentor Support):

People need support at all stages of their recovery. You can speak to Joe himself about that through his Quad-Rebuild charity, and the Spinal Injuries Association can also link you with the right people at the right time to help you move on in life. There are options out there for you, whether that is counselling or peer-level support. People inevitably think it's counselling that they need, but sometimes, it's just speaking to somebody else who understands. I have found time and time again, that speaking to a peer can really help. As will reading this book. Getting in touch can lead you in so many different ways and open up so many avenues of help and support.

The SIA also has regional groups where spinal cord injured people can get together – and that definitely includes family and friends – so they can chat to people and learn from each other. From my sports days, I know how empowering it is to be with a group who really understand each other.

Joe:

Whether you find that help with a psychologist or a spinal injury group, you can find a way to put the past behind you without resentment. You don't have to bury the past, but you do have to come to terms with it because the quicker you move beyond it, the quicker you can start to rebuild your life. That's why our charity's motto is *rebuilding lives*. I know what you've been through, I was there too. That is why I want you to know that don't have to come to terms with it on your own. We are here to help you.

It isn't always easy. I couldn't find that direction until I had reached a place of acceptance. But I found out that having a direction or a sense of purpose is important. You need to find that thing that will bring you happiness or contentment. Having something to focus on, no matter how big or small can help you start again.

Now, I feel energised and passionate about the new future that I want to create for myself. I feel as if I have been given an opportunity to help so many other people, and I am compelled to do that. I have a clear direction, and while I still want to be involved in construction work, I want to follow my vocation to help people. I want to be able to look back when I'm older and be satisfied with my achievements.

I think that is the secret to a good life, whoever you are. You need to keep striving...

Andy (Mentor Support):

In time I realised that I wanted a little bit more out of life, I wanted to find fulfilling work and settle down. I met my partner who is now my wife. I couldn't ever have imagined it in my darkest days, but now, I have a wife and two daughters, I work four days a week, nine-to-five, I drive, I go on holiday, I drop the kids off at school; I really live a very average life! Which is, of course, an extraordinary thing.

Joe:

I do want to take some more time for myself to do meaningful things and to meet new people. I do want to make a future with somebody. The specialists tell me that because I breathe with a ventilator, I have a lower life expectancy, but their estimates are based on current statistics, and it gives me yet another reason to want to eat healthily and stay as active as I can.

Kate (Joe's Friend):

We have all seen how it's important to believe in what's still possible. I know that Joe is really keen to meet somebody special and embark on a new relationship. It's very easy for him to assume that it will never happen, but the world has changed so much. There are all sorts of dating sites out there for all sorts of people. He can definitely still meet somebody.

Sam (Joe's Sister):

I've spoken to Joe about the future, and I always say, nothing's impossible. Joe has spoken about how much he'd like to have another relationship, and a family... Who's to say he can't have those things? If you want that, you can go out there and get it.

There are options for parenting too, for surrogates, and nannies; the way we think about what he can achieve has changed. The future he can have won't be the future he would have had, but it can still give him so much of what he wants from life. He's young enough to make a whole new life for himself.

Joe:

I've always wanted a family of my own, and I still cherish that dream. If I met somebody who would want to go on that journey with me, it would bring a real emotional depth back into my life. Dating after a life-changing accident shouldn't be impossible, but it does come with challenges. I've been on several different websites that include people with disabilities, but some of the definitions of disability are a bit different to what you or I may be experiencing! I have searched the web extensively and have not yet found any dating websites that have specialised in people with spinal cord injuries. I think the only way forward is for me to create one.

Having a physically affectionate relationship with someone may not be possible in the same way for me, or perhaps for you, but companionship – having someone to share our lives with – is so important. No offence to all my carers – I love them all to bits – but it would be nice to have a more significant relationship with someone. I'm resilient enough to know that it might not happen, but that doesn't stop me looking.

Timing is important. I wouldn't have been ready for a relationship for quite a long time. I was still in mourning for the relationship I had lost. You can't move on until you've got over the hurdles of a past relationship, or past the change that your injury has brought to your life. But you will know when the time is right for you. I think there is someone out there for me, and I'm excited for the future…

18 The Love and Support of Friends and Family

The effectiveness of any recovery process can be greatly enhanced by your network of friends and family. There may need to be adjustments, but you don't have to reframe your relationships with them; you just need to stick together and help each other.

> *When you can't reassure someone anymore – because there are times when that isn't going to work – you just listen. You don't even need to say anything. You just need to be there on the end of the phone, or in person and just listen.*

Kate (Joe's Friend):

Joe knows that everybody is really proud of him, he knows we're all there for him, but there will be days when he doesn't want to get out of bed and face the world. There must be times when everything feels pretty dark.

Joe:

It upsets me that I sometimes feel lonely. I feel as if I don't deserve that. Yes, I have a large family around me that loves me, but that doesn't take away from the fact that I can feel isolated and alone sometimes. I have had to accept that the people that I care about have their own lives to lead, they have to earn a living, or care for their immediate families. It hurts sometimes if I feel alone on a Saturday night, and I just want to be able to cuddle up to someone and watch a film.

But I also know that I can do something about it. I will reach out to my family and tell them if I feel lonely. Sometimes I'll call one of my sisters and tell them that I don't want to be in on my own, and they are always happy to come and spend some time with me. You have to feel able to reach out to the people you care about.

Michaela (Joe's Sister):

We tried to help him together. If he rang me, I'd ring my other sister afterwards and ask her to speak to him too. And when you can't

DOI: 10.4324/9781003430728-21

reassure someone anymore – because there are times when reassurance isn't going to work – you just listen. You don't even need to say anything. You just need to be there on the end of the phone, or in person and just listen.

It was usually at night when the anxiety set in. And when he used to feel like that, and he was so desperate and crying his eyes out, all we could do was to tell him, *Joe, we know you can do it, because you already are doing it.*

Kate (Joe's Friend):

There are times when he puts on a front for everybody; he doesn't want people to know that he's struggling, but I know that he still has his bad days. Sometimes he'll message me and say he can't deal with it, or he'll tell me that he's struggling.

In those times, I think he really just wants somebody to talk to. He wants to tell people how he's feeling. Of course, he has his carers around him all the time, but sometimes he needs to talk to his friends about what's really going on for him. I think sometimes he wants some reassurance. He works so hard at reassuring others that he needs some reassurance back in return. You can tell someone you're there for them as many times as you want, but that isn't going to stop them from feeling lonely sometimes. And there isn't always something that anybody can do to take that level of loneliness away. It isn't about what I can say to Joe sometimes; it's just about being there for him.

Joe:

Perhaps you're reading this, and you feel isolated and lonely too. Perhaps you don't have family or friends to call in on you. Even if you are used to being the most independent person, it can be hard to adjust to a lonelier life. I'm not saying the loneliness will ever go away, but I do believe that it can be managed. I think that the more socialising you can do, the better. Even if it feels like a struggle at first, it does help. There are spinal injury groups and associations where you can meet other people and talk about your experiences with people who really understand what you're going through. You might even meet a special someone; you'll almost certainly make friends.

Kate (Joe's Friend):

If you're a friend of someone like Joe, the best thing you can do is to just be there for them, and be as positive as you can. There were numerous times when Joe got locked in a negative mindset, and it was important for us to try and get him out of that. It's not about lying or being over-optimistic, it's just about reminding them of the things that are possible and practical.

Barry (Joe's Friend):

If I could go back and give myself some advice before I took the phone call from Michelle telling me that Joe had been in a terrible accident, and he might not pull through, it would simply be: *This is going to take time. Be patient.*

Normally, when somebody is injured, they get better. Whether they've broken an arm or a leg, you put a splint on it, or plaster, and in a few weeks, they're in physiotherapy. A few weeks after that, they're right as rain. But when something like this happens, something catastrophic, you need to have all the patience in the world, both with yourself and the person that's in recovery.

I'd have told myself, your sympathy doesn't really help. Joe doesn't need your sympathy, he needs you to work on understanding what he's trying to say or do. You are going to have to try to understand how he's feeling. Be empathetic, not sympathetic.

Feeling sorry for somebody can be as bad as wounding them all over again. You're sorry because they're broken. Nobody wants that. You have to be a shining beacon for them. And that doesn't mean trying to do everything for them. You may think that you're helping, but if you do too much, it probably won't help. There's a fine line between helping and running someone's life for them. You need to try and be aware of where that line is, and be mindful of the fact that it moves like the tide. What you do one day may feel like too much the next day.

Michaela (Joe's Sister):

Joe's get-up-and-go is still there. His determination to make something of his life is still there. That's why he's done a university degree, and he's working hard to help people who experience what he did. He really wants to help people understand – to feel what it's like to go through it. I won't ever know how Joseph actually feels, but I know how it feels to go through it as part of Joe's family.

Joe:

I am hard on myself sometimes, but it's almost ingrained in me. That's how I've always been. And I've come through all of this wanting to show people that life is there to be lived. Perhaps there have been times where I have tried to achieve too much, even at the expense of my own happiness. I don't know how to wind down. I do like to make other people happy, and that makes me happy.

Sam (Joe's Sister):

He's done so well, he's been amazing really, but it must be hard for him to see that. So many people would have given up after just some of the challenges he's faced, but Joe never has.

You can't keep Joe down. He signed up for uni, and started his Quad-Rebuild charity. His drive was still there, and he found other things to do. He found other outlets for his energy, and it helped keep that drive going.

Michaela (Joe's Sister):

I think his determination has always pulled us through, and it's been a lot longer now since he rang one of us to say he couldn't do it anymore.

Kate (Joe's Friend):

The positivity in him is amazing. The fact that he managed to keep himself so busy was such a big factor in his recovery. It helped him focus on something else. There have been times when he's been poorly and ended up in hospital, and it isn't the illness that brings him down, it's the fact that he can't go to uni, or he can't do his work. That's when he has too much time on his hands to think about things.

Joe has always said throughout the time since the accident, I need visitors, I need to see my friends. And I think it's so important to keep those friendships going.

Ross (Joe's Friend):

He doesn't speak about what he's going through very much. Sometimes he'll just say 'it's shit,' but he'd much rather have a laugh and carry on as close to where we were before as we can.

Kate (Joe's Friend):

There are challenges to maintaining a friendship after an event like this. I think here may have been times when Joe has been aware of some of his friends going out and if he's not been invited, it's very easy for him to feel left out. But in those situations, I'll remind him that even as an able-bodied person you don't get invited out all the time. People have different friendship groups and there are times when life doesn't revolve around you! I certainly don't get invited everywhere, so there have been times when I have to bring him back down to earth.

I do still feel some of that same heartbreak when I've been with him – knowing what he's lost. What happened to him hasn't happened to me, or to any of our friends, and I cannot imagine how he's feeling. So, I do struggle when he's having a bad day, because I don't always understand what's going on underneath.

Ross (Joe's Friend):

> The strange thing about Joe is that when you're with him, you can almost forget. I see him sometimes and we have a chat and then half an hour later, it hits me. That's his life now.

Kate (Joe's Friend):

> In spite of everything that has happened, I feel as if our friendship is actually better than ever. Life gets in the way of friendships sometimes, but since his accident, I feel as if I've seen Joe more often, and it feels as if we're closer. And I think that's the case with some of his other friends too. I think that Joe has lost some of his friendships because of his changed circumstances, but he really values his close friends, the ones who've stuck with him. We all release how close we were to losing Joe. That certainly brings you closer together. We're lucky that he didn't pass away, and we know we need to make the most of our friendships.

Ross (Joe's Friend):

> Whenever we go out together, it's like rolling back the years in a way. Everything feels normal. We can chat about life in general, and what we're going to do next. So maybe that's the secret: even after everything that's happened, that person is still your son, your daughter, your friend, or your partner, and your relationship with them can carry on. That's when you know that nothing can stop your relationship

Kate (Joe's Friend):

> Joe has really valued being able to go out with us when he can. And I'm sure that's true for anyone who has had to adjust to spending so much of their life at home after an accident or illness. We plan plenty of days out and meals out. I want to be there for him as and when he needs me.
>
> I still feel that sadness around what he's lost, but more than ever, I just feel proud of him for everything he's done. If it had been me, I don't think I'd have been able to do any of the things that he has done, and that he's continuing to do. He's still doing so many amazing things. I would never pity him; I look at what he's doing and he's doing really well for himself.

Joe:

> It isn't just you that needs to accept change; it's the people you live with, your family and friends.
>
> Not everyone is going to be able to go with you on your journey because not everyone is going to be able to make the right kind of adjustment. My real friends and my family understand that.

People will have different opinions about the right way forward for you; they will think differently. But you can't control that. In the early days, I lashed out at people when they disagreed with me, but I had to learn to let that go. Through my distress tolerance work I have learned that I can only control what I say, I can't control any outcomes, and I can't control what anyone else says.

The changes you have to make in your life, and the path that you decide upon will almost certainly be met by resistance from some people. A lot of the work you do is in adjusting your mindset, but another massive part of the work you'll need to do is help the people around you to adjust their mindsets too. Not everyone is going to respond in the same way to you after your accident or illness. Some of them might think they have all the answers to help you. You might even find that some people can't join you on the journey you're taking. Some people will always think they know better, and some will think your decisions are the wrong ones. The one thing you have to do more than anything else is: be true to yourself. This is your injury, your rehabilitation, and your life.

It's also worth remembering that your family and friends won't have had the same sort of psychological support in dealing with what has happened that you have hopefully had. Before I did any EMDR and before I had any counselling, I would rage at my situation, I would hurl nasty words at everyone. I need to remember what it used to be like for me before I had EMDR and stress tolerance techniques to help me understand how to control my body, my mind, and my actions so that I could articulate what I wanted and needed.

Manage what goes on in your head and what comes out of your mouth instead of trying to control what other people think and say. You'll never be able to influence or control what anyone else thinks or says anyway, so you need to be able to let that go. There is no good in harbouring any resentment, or stressing about the fact that your friends or family can't always see your world through your eyes. Just try to accept it. Just concentrate on managing your own responses to situations, not on trying to control what anybody else says or does.

Kate (Joe's Friend):

When I think about how he looked, and how he was back then, there has been such a massive change in him. He doesn't always see it that way. But for me, having seen him in that bed when he was in such a bad state, seeing the change in him now is incredible. He's achieved so much in such a short space of time. He's so strong-willed and positive now.

Joe:

I do feel as if this has happened for a reason, and that has helped me to accept my body and my limitations. I am comfortable in my own skin, and I'm comfortable with the way I look. The sooner you can recognise the restrictions that face you, the better. This is a central part of rehabilitation.

Andy (Mentor Support):

Let's not forget, it's still relatively early days for Joe. He still needs support, because of the level of injury he sustained, he will always need support, but he can also go on and continue to achieve remarkable things. But the way he has dealt with it all has been amazing. Joe means a lot to me; and he never fails to impress me with his resilience.

Joe:

Learning to let go, and letting resentment melt away is key. And that's why having the support of psychologists and other therapists is so helpful. I know there are people, out there who can't access those services, and that's why I want to pass on what I've learned to them through Quad-Rebuild.

Paul (Joe's Brother):

I go and see Joe whenever I can. I'll always be there for him. If he ever needs anything doing, I'll do it. We can talk about pretty much anything, but apart from that one time, we've not really talked about the accident. Maybe we still will. Maybe we should.

The one important message I can offer you if you're reading this and your life has been changed like mine was – and like Joe's was – is don't give up. My brother proves what is possible. Even though he can only move his head, he's doing things that most normal people can't do. He needs help to do lots of things, but he's shown us that you should never give up on yourself. I can't believe how he gets up and carries on every day; he's strong and he never gives up on himself.

Even if you can't move, I know that things can change, and things can be done to help.

Mary (Joe's Mum):

I want Joe to have a happy life. I know that he will be successful in his business. He's already done so many things the doctors said he'd never be able to do. He's got his uni course, and he's thinking about podcasting. I'd like to think he will have the family he wants; he's spoken about IVF. He won't ever be left on his own. Even if it isn't me, or it isn't his dad, this family will be there for him. He loves the family getting together.

Michaela (Joe's Sister):

I know were not the first family to go through this, and we won't be the last. But I hope that it helps people to know that even when times are tough and life feels darker than it has ever felt before, you can get through it. There may be times when it feels impossible, but day-by day, hour-by-hour, or minute-by-minute if you have to, you can get through it.

It's funny how quickly your lives adapt to your new circumstances. When we get together now, we just talk about the normal everyday things. The practical things have changed. Joe is a typical man, but he has been able to talk to us a little bit about how he's really feeling, and it's important that he can do that.

Mary (Joe's Mum):

He still talks to me about whatever he needs to talk about. And when things have been really tough, we can talk things through as a family too.

Sam (Joe's Sister):

We've always been close as brothers and sisters. So it didn't matter what he said to us when he was feeling frustrated. It didn't matter how rude he might have been, because we all knew where that frustration was coming from, and we weren't going to fall out with him over it.

That didn't mean we'd just take it. I was perfectly happy to say, "No, I'm not listening to that." Our relationship didn't really change at all in that respect.

Barry (Joe's Friend):

I consider Joe a really good mate, but I'm old enough to be his dad. Joe loves his own dad very much, but I knew that he felt comfortable enough to talk to me in ways he maybe couldn't talk to some of his younger friends. Before he was injured, Joe could sometimes put on a bit of bravado for his mates. But he was always honest about how he was feeling with me. He's grown less afraid of opening up, and that has really helped him.

Michaela (Joe's Sister):

Nobody would have asked for what happened to happen, but there are some positives. Above all, I'm thankful that Joe is still alive – we were having to face the prospect of losing him, and we're so relieved that his brain was okay. We see each other more now than we used to. We all have our own lives, and he used to work all hours of the day, so we only used to see each other on special occasions. But now, we make the time, and I see him a lot more, we all do. We go out for breakfast or lunch now, and it's been nice to have those little moments of connection which we didn't have before.

Sam (Joe's Sister):

Above all, you have to try and keep your faith and hang on in there. Life may not be the same again afterwards, but things can get better. Our family pulled together for Joe, and it's wonderful how people really do rally round and try and help however they can.

19   A Remarkable Journey

Recovery was too small an aim for Joe. Since his accident, he has been working towards a higher aim of post-traumatic growth; of achieving more than anyone ever thought possible.

Never give up hope. Life isn't over. This is your new life. And it is a second chance.

Joe:

>I've lost count of the number of times people will say to me *you can't do that!* A good example is going on holiday. When I was planning to go on holiday last, one of my carers was scared to do it. They hadn't cared for me outside of the house before, and I reminded them they'd never changed a tracheostomy before, but they'd learned how to do that.
>
>Having a spinal cord injury obviously puts restrictions on where you can go and what you can do, but it shouldn't restrict your goals, aspirations, and dreams. It shouldn't stop you doing what you want to do. Stare those problems in the face and challenge your demons.

Mary (Joe's Mum):

>Joe loves going on holiday – he's been to all sorts of places since his accident. Although it's difficult because he needs six carers with him – but we all rally round, and we organise things so that everyone can get together.

Michaela (Joe's Sister):

>Joe has done so much they said he wouldn't be able to do. We are all super-proud of him, and of everything that he does. Even now, today, four years later, it's hard. Sometimes *I look at him and think if only things had been different*. He'd be in his happy marriage now. I think he would have had his big business by now. He always had that big determination, and he would have made his ambitions happen.

DOI: 10.4324/9781003430728-22

But Joe is so much better now than he was. We know he won't ever be the same again, but slowly and surely, we've been getting him back – the son, brother, and friend that we knew and loved.

Katherine (Neuropsychologist):

I know that a lot of post-traumatic growth can – and does – happen. It can take a little longer, but I have worked with many people who go on to have an entirely different appreciation of life. They forge different relationships with people. They see new possibilities in life. They focus more on their own personal strengths. There can be spiritual change. At the start of the journey, I know that the idea of that kind of growth might seem absurd. And it certainly isn't something that we would normally discuss until somebody's psychological scaffolding is firmly entrenched. But as people move along, I have seen that a natural information processing action seems to happen that helps us adapt.

In a recent session with Joe, we were talking about life values, and he said that he would never have ascribed as much value to relationships as he does now. He finds that now that he has switched off from work a little bit more, he feels lonely, and he realises that he wants to forge relationships. The motivation for him to do that hasn't just appeared suddenly, like so many parts of the process, it has grown in him to the point that he now wants to make a change. Before the accident, those thoughts just wouldn't have occurred to him.

Joe:

The way that I treat people, the way that I communicate with them, has changed. I make sure that people know how much I value and appreciate them. Being positive with people, even if they are making me feel frustrated or angry is the best way to deal with any situation. It's certainly the best way to get the most out of any relationship at work. I wish I'd understood that earlier in life!

Katie (Case Manager):

The journey with Joe has been remarkable in many ways. His enthusiasm for his goals in life has not wavered. He has stayed consistent in what he wants to achieve, despite clinical and health setbacks along the way. Joe has had some significant hospital admissions, but always comes back with the same ideas and enthusiasm.

Joe:

Right from the start, I knew I could use my experience to try and help others. With Quad-Rebuild, we are building a community. It's a family. All of us have been through this injury, and we can all help each other and be there for each other. Quad-Rebuild will help to bring us all together.

Barry (Joe's Friend):

He's inspirational. Joe could hardly write when I met him, now he's done a degree course!

I understand why he needs to do things. I'm retired and I need my projects, and Joe has so much left to give. He started Quad-Rebuild because he wanted to help people see that there is still light at the end of the tunnel. He's a beacon of light and hope.

Joe:

People may find it hard to believe, but in a weird way, I'm glad that this accident happened to me. I'm glad that it's put me in this position, it has helped me find my vocation in life: Quad-Rebuild…

Katie (Case Manager)

Despite the physical and emotional difficulties, Joe is absolutely unwavering in terms of what he wants to achieve. In large part, that is because Joe never just thinks about himself; he is deeply committed to his charity endeavours. So, if he has a difficult experience, he won't just think about that from his own point of view, he'll think about how it might impact somebody else. He wants to try and ensure that other people don't have to experience the same kinds of avoidable issues, by learning from his experience. He always sees the bigger picture, both in terms of his own life to come, and in terms of people like him, and helping make their experience better.

Sam (Joe's Sister):

Most of all, he wants to go on helping others. We quickly found out that there isn't a lot out there for people with his injuries for the simple reason that people don't often survive that kind of incident. Every part of his life was affected, and everything needed its own solution. For example, he can't use his hands so we had to try and find a cup with a long straw so that when he's thirsty he can have a drink without having to wait for somebody to help him. He needed special support for his iPad so he could go on using it, and something he could comfortably hold in his mouth to type. We found tools and resources for paraplegics, but not very much for people like Joe. So that only convinced him how much more he could do to help people learn from his experience.

Joe:

I was in the last four months of my rehab, and I was still with Michelle. Andy Wharton from the Spinal Injuries Association knocked on my door one day and told me about his work. After a few sessions with him I felt as if something was missing. I wanted to know why there wasn't the same kind of support for quadriplegics. Why wasn't anyone going around helping people like me? That was the first trigger.

The next thing was seeing people in hospital who had been there for a year, a year and a half, or even longer. They couldn't leave because some of them had to sell their house, or get major renovations done before they could move back. So many of them were waiting for some sort of social housing, or waiting for a space in a nursing home. I wanted to know why there wasn't something out there to help people make that move back home, or make the adaptations they needed.

I talked to more and more people about the problems, and about the need for a charity. That's when one of my friends said, so why don't you create one? I had already been thinking about making house adaptations, but I knew that many people wouldn't be able to afford them; I knew it needed to be a charity.

Quad-Rebuild is here to help people in lots of ways. Sometimes that will be about rebuilding their image. When I saw people in hospital with me, I sometimes thought how scruffy they looked, or how ill-kempt, little realising that I looked just the same. That struck me as wrong. Just because we'd been injured, it didn't mean that we had to let everything else go.

I've been lucky to have the correct support, and I think that's vital for anybody with a spinal cord injury. The timing of it is important too. It isn't the right time to worry about these things when you're in hospital, you need that time to rehabilitate your body and work on your psychological state. But when you get out of hospital, you are probably going to need more support, and that's where Quad-Rebuild comes in.

Our motto sums it up: Rebuilding homes. Rebuild your image. Rebuilding the future.

Speaking to people in hospital and on forums, I knew there were so many things that could and should be done to help people with spinal injuries. We'll be collaborating with other charities to help as many people in as many ways as we can. In particular, we'll specialise in house adaptations because there's no one else who does that.

Most of all, we need a community. Quad-Rebuild exists to help people get together and share experiences, or get out on trips to re-open our eyes to the world. I knew how important it is for people to get back to doing some of the things they used to do – getting out to pubs, clubs and restaurants, and getting out on holiday. Just going shopping, or getting a haircut, these little things are an important part of our daily lives.

We're starting in Sheffield and Leeds Pinderfields – it's where I was reborn, after all. After that, we're hoping to expand to Stoke Mandeville en route to becoming a national charity – that's the aim. We're all working towards the dream of having quad centres up and down the country to give help wherever it's needed. We're looking to draft in volunteers to help us, and recruiting and training mentors and other helpers.

There's a wider message too. I want to get out to schools and universities, and speak to all sorts of people. I want to be a part of those campaigns to remind people what can happen if they don't wear a seatbelt, or they don't take breaks when they're driving. I want to create and share presentations to show people that life is worth living, to never give up on your hopes and dreams, regardless of your situation. I want to take Paul with me and go into schools, colleges, hospitals, prisons, anywhere and everywhere, and I want to tell them, *show* them what happens.

It doesn't just have to be about spinal injuries. I think my story shows that just because something happens to you – and it doesn't even matter what it is – it doesn't mean that your life is over. People who are in prison can still make something of their lives. People who have put on weight, or failed at something, or survived something terrible can still rise above all of that. You can still have a fulfilling life if you change the path you've been on.

Speaking to people with spinal injuries will be my main focus though. I want to be able to talk to them in very real and raw terms about my life and what I've learnt along the way. And there is one message that rings out loud and clear:

Never give up hope. Life isn't over. This is your new life. And it is a second chance. You've got this!

Afterword

As I write this, five years after the accident, I most definitely look at life in a completely different way. That does not mean to say it is a good or bad thing that has happened to me; I believe that events like this are a part of life that some of us must accept regardless of how careful we are. My family has had to deal with a lot, and by that I don't just mean the injury, I mean the arguments, and all the times I projected my feelings in an unhelpful way by shouting and screaming at them. Your family will be going through the exact same things that mine were. They are struggling too, they just might not show it, so they can be strong for you. Remember that there is a lack of awareness and conversation around issues like paralysis and quadriplegia. Do not underestimate how little people know about spinal cord injuries until it happens to someone they know.

Some people will get upset with you, it is so hard for them to understand what you are going through at that moment in time, but do remember that they love you. They want to help you in any way they can, and they will, without a doubt, feel helpless. It will take time for them to get used to you living a new life in a wheelchair. Others will have the understanding that you have just been through one of the biggest catastrophic life-changing injuries anyone can ever experience. They are there for you no matter what, and they understand the level of support you need. Sometimes, just being by your side through thick and thin is all it takes.

Try not to push people away, they just want to be with you while you are suffering, sharing those pains and experiences. Some of course, back away, they feel helpless, and it is such a difficult thing for some people to watch another human being go through an experience like this. Don't you always wonder how people come in and out of your life at different times? Well, one thing I am sure you will already know by now is that people will fall out of your life when you thought that they would be there for you more than others. And people that wouldn't normally be there, will step up and show their support. It's so easy to think negatively when you are experiencing such a life changing injury. Keeping focussed to concentrate on your rehabilitation is one of the fundamental keys to understanding your injury and rebuilding a positive state of mind.

The specialists in the spinal units will be instrumental in helping you learn about spinal injuries and all the things you must do to look after your body. It is extremely important to follow the guidelines that the rehab units set in place to help you manage your injury. The extent of your injury will determine the level of care you need. Most paraplegics will discharge from a spinal unit without needing care in the community. The higher your level of spinal break and amount of mobility you have does determine whether you need one-to-one care or two-to-one care. Furthermore, if you are ventilated then this can affect the decision of whether or not you have two waking carers all night, or one waking and one sleeping. Reaching a point where you feel you're at peace with your carers can be extremely difficult. You may be upset one day and your carers may not be considerate to your needs, but it is all about taking the rough with the smooth. In the early days, you will find it difficult, and you may have moments of feeling like you don't want to be here anymore. Be honest about your feelings, take all the love, care, and support that is out there for you, and hold on.

Looking back on my experiences – and especially when I think back to when I was first discharged from hospital – I wasn't a very nice person. I mean, who would be when they have just had their life turned upside down and all their dreams shattered? I can say for sure though, if I could turn back time I wouldn't be that same person again. One thing that my friend always tries to teach me, "Is that really going to bother you tomorrow or next week, because if it isn't then let it go." That is me now, saying those words to my younger self. I now treat my carers like my family and I wouldn't have it any other way. If I have learnt one thing over the last few years, it is to treat people how you would like to be treated.

To sum everything up, I am just a man in a broken body. The only difference is that I am a wheelchair user. Do you really think that just because you are in a wheelchair, you should let that hold you back? No, I don't think it should. If you don't agree with me, then it is my prerogative to come and work with you, to support you. Whether you are reading this as a friend, family member, or the person at the epicentre of the injury, I am here to show you that regardless of the disability, life is for living. Every cloud has a silver lining, and it is about finding the way forward that works for you. You have read my journey, and now it's my turn to learn about yours.

Joe

Appendix 1
Organisations That Can Help You

There is a small selection of charities that support spinal cord injuries:

Quad-Rebuild

Joe's own charity, offering a complete package of advice, support, and practical assistance. The charities' four mottos show how they can help you:

Rebuilding Lives

At Quad-rebuild we create a bespoke plan for you. Assisting, supporting, and advising you on what to expect is vital for your rehabilitation.

Rebuilding Homes

Coming from a background in building helped Joe to realise how he could support people in their community by providing grants to adapt your home. Aiding you to move around your home independently is a key building block to improving mental health.

Rebuilding Your Image

Coming to terms with your injury and working on your self-acceptance, self-image, and self-confidence is fundamental to rebuilding your life.

Rebuilding Your Future

Helping you to move from rehabilitation and into your home, building on confidence to live an active normal life is a fundamental part of your transition back into society.

www.quad-rebuild.co.uk

Spinal Injuries Association

Experts in care management services and consumable delivery.
    https://www.spinal.co.uk

Back Up

The Back Up Trust challenges you to achieve new goals and provides support and mentoring.
    https://www.backuptrust.org.uk

Aspire

Providing support-assistive technology advice, temporary housing, benefits advice, and help with independent living.
    https://www.aspire.org.uk

Day One

For professional services to help anyone affected by major trauma, including psychological intervention, legal support, benefits and welfare advice, and emergency funding.
    https://www.dayonetrauma.org

Benefits and Entitlements

You may be entitled to claim for benefits and/or support, including the following:

- Universal credit
- Personal independence payments (PIPs)
- Housing benefit
- Council tax benefit
- Disabled facility grants from charities.

You can apply for grants from Quad-Rebuild for:

- Travel and accommodation (to help you see your loved ones while you're in rehabilitation).
- Adapting your home.
- Providing equipment to make you more independent, including eyegaze computers, iPads, stands, and mouth sticks.

Appendix 2
A Basic Introduction to Spinal Injuries

What Is a Spinal Cord?

The spinal cord is a network of nerves that run from the brain's base and down the length of your back within your spine. The spinal cord is protected by spinal fluid and the bones of the spine which are called vertebrae. The nerve fibres send messages to the brain which then send messages to the rest of the body, these messages may be for movement, sensation, feeling, or pain.

What Is a Spinal Cord Injury?

A spinal cord injury (SCI) is when damage occurs to the spinal cord, through illness or trauma at any level of the spine. This results in change which is either temporary or permanent in the normal motor, sensory, or autonomic function of the cord.

If the spinal cord is damaged, the signals that go between our brain and the rest of the body can't get through. This results in a loss of movement and sensation from below the level of injury.

There are many different reasons a SCI can occur, but the most common causes of a SCI include the following:

- Road traffic accidents
- Falls
- Sports injuries
- Violence inflicted injuries

There are two main types of SCI, known as 'complete' and 'incomplete'.

Complete SCI is the most severe. In these cases, there is enough trauma to cause damage across the whole width of the spinal cord which results in a complete and permanent loss of function and sensation below the level of injury.

Incomplete SCI is more common. In these cases, areas of the spinal cord remain intact, meaning that instead of a complete loss of function, some mobility and sensation will remain.

Different Levels of Injury and What Movement Can Be Lost

The higher the injury on the spinal cord, the more loss can occur.

High cervical (C1–C4)
- May have paralysis in arms, hands, trunk, and legs. When all four limbs are affected, this is called quadriplegia or tetraplegia.
- May not be able to breathe on his or her own, cough, or control bladder and bowel movements.
- Speaking is sometimes impaired or reduced.

Low cervical (C5–C8)
- May have paralysis in hands, trunk, and legs.
- With this level of injury, a person may be able to breathe on their own and speak normally.

Thoracic (T1–T5)
- May have paralysis in trunk and legs.
- Usually affect the chest, abdominal, mid-back muscles, and legs.
- Have normal hand, arm, and upper body movement.

Thoracic (T6–T12)
- May have paralysis in trunk and legs
- Usually affect the abdominal, lower back muscles, and legs.
- Will have normal hand, arm, and upper body movement.

Lumber (L1–L5)
- Usually results in some loss of function to the hips and legs.
- Depending on the strength of legs, may need to use a wheelchair or use leg braces.

Sacral (S1–S5)
- May result in some loss of function in the hips or legs.
- Someone with this level of injury will most likely be able to walk.

Side Effects of a Spinal Cord Injury

Autonomic Dysreflexia (AD)

Not everyone will suffer from AD but this can occur in individuals with a SCI at level T6 and above. It is an abnormal overreaction of the involuntary (autonomic) nervous system to stimulation. The reaction may include change in heart rate, high blood pressure, excessive sweating, muscle spasms, headache, and change in skin colour (paleness, redness, blue/grey tinge colour). Bladder issues are the most common trigger of AD. Bowel and some skin conditions can also cause AD.

Hypotension

Low blood pressure, also called hypotension, is when the pressure in your blood vessels is unusually low. Symptoms of low blood pressure can include dizziness, feeling sick, and fainting.

Treatment for low blood pressure will depend on what's causing it. It might involve things like wearing support stockings or drinking more water.

Causes of low blood pressure include ageing, pregnancy, and some medical conditions or medicines.

Chest Infections

Cervical and thoracic SCI's can weaken the chest and abdominal muscles resulting in respiratory infections such as common cold, flu, and pneumonia.

Pressure Sores

Pressure sores can occur due to reduced movement which is why it is important to have regular pressure relief and to be turned regularly when immobile in bed for long periods of time. It is important to seek treatment immediately for pressure sores as they can quickly become infected.

Bladder and Bowel Issues

A SCI sometimes interrupts communication between the brain and the nerves in the spinal cord that control bladder and bowel function. This can cause bladder and bowel dysfunction known as neurogenic bladder or neurogenic bowel. People with multiple sclerosis or spina bifida might have similar problems.

Signs and symptoms of neurogenic bladder may include the following:
- Loss of bladder control
- Inability to empty the bladder
- Urinary frequency
- Urinary tract infections

Signs of neurogenic bowel include the following:
- Loss of bowel control
- Constipation
- Bowel frequency
- Lack of bowel movements

There are treatment options and other ways to manage your bladder and bowel which should be discussed with your medical professionals.

Your Mental Health and Wellbeing

A big number of SCI's are due to a major/catastrophic event, and as a result, an individual will have to face a new way of life which can be mentally and emotionally challenging. Accepting changes to life, untreated distress, grief/loss around loss of previous life and relationships takes time. It is important to speak to professionals/family/friends to help you accept your new way of life and all the challenges you may face.

Index